Borderline Personality Disorder

A survival guide to BPD, mood swings, and personality disorders

Table of Contents

Introduction 1

Chapter 1: What Is Borderline Personality Disorder? 2

Chapter 2: Symptoms of Borderline Personality Disorder 11

Chapter 3: Diagnosis of Borderline Personality Disorder 16

Chapter 4: Brain Function of a Person with BPD 20

Chapter 5: What Happens During a BPD Episode 24

Chapter 6: Treatments for Borderline Personality Disorder ... 28

Chapter 7: Finding the Right Therapist 39

Chapter 8: Lifestyle Treatment Methods 47

Chapter 9: Self Help Strategies During an Episode 57

Chapter 10: Exercises for BPD 67

Chapter 11: Meditation for BPD 69

Chapter 12: Borderline Personality Disorder at Work and School 86

Chapter 13: Helping a Loved One with BPD 92

Chapter 14: Borderline Personality Disorder FAQs 104

Chapter 15: Can People with BPD Succeed in Life? 111

Conclusion 114

Introduction

Thank you for taking the time to read this book on Borderline Personality Disorder.

This book covers the topic of Borderline Personality Disorder, and will educate you on the different signs and symptoms of BPD.

Throughout the following chapters, you will discover how BPD is diagnosed, the different treatment methods available, self-help strategies you can implement, and ways that you can help a loved one with BPD.

Borderline Personality Disorder can have a huge impact on a person's life in many different ways. It can affect their work life, their relationships, and their overall wellbeing. However, it doesn't have to totally control a person. This book will provide you with steps and strategies to control BPD symptoms, and maintain a normal healthy lifestyle, despite a BPD diagnosis.

Once again, thanks for choosing this book, I hope you find it to be helpful!

Chapter 1: What Is Borderline Personality Disorder?

Borderline Personality Disorder, or BPD, is a mental health disorder that affects your relationship with yourself and with other people. It is often characterized by a distorted self-image, impulsiveness, extreme emotions, and intense relationships.

People diagnosed with BPD often suffer through a mix of intense emotions that can be anywhere from extremely good to extremely bad. Individuals with BPD may have a fear of abandonment, be unstable emotionally, and veer towards anger and impulsiveness at inappropriate times.

Of course, all people experience intense emotions at some point in their life. People with BPD, however, have a long-term pattern of such behavior with no known triggers, or very "soft" triggers. Simply put, those with BPD can have episodes for reasons that would not normally trigger intense emotions in other people.

The variety of intense emotions is often just the jump off point of the disorder. As a result of these feelings, people with BPD can turn suicidal, engage in self-harm, experience depression, suffer from anxiety, become alcoholics, take drugs, or participate in many other self-destructive activities.

Population of BPD
Studies show that around 1.6 percent of people are diagnosed with BPD every year, with women being diagnosed with the condition 3 times as often as men. Of course, this can be because men are less likely to seek help if they think they're suffering from any form of mental disorder. Despite the seriousness of the condition, BPD sadly still has a stigma attached to it.

Here are some additional quick statistics on Borderline Personality Disorder:

- BPD is actually more common than schizophrenia

- Surface records reveal that around 2 percent of the general public have BPD. Further studies, however, show that the numbers are much higher than that, reaching as much as 5.9 percent, equally divided between genders.

- BPD is actually twice as common as anorexia.

- Around 33 percent of young people committing suicide shows symptoms of BPD. Around 10 percent of adults who commit suicide are diagnosed with Borderline Personality.

- A person with BPD is 400 times more likely to commit suicide.

- Currently, there is no FDA-approved medication directly targeting BPD.

- Around 40 percent of mental health service users are diagnosed with BPD.

- More than 50 percent of people with BPD are not employable or are impaired in their likelihood of employment.

- Around 28 percent of women in prison have BPD. while 12 percent of the men are diagnosed with the condition.

How the Public Views BPD

There are still negative connotations attached to BPD, and a divided belief system with respect to the condition. This isn't really surprising considering that mental health problems are still being studied, and treatments for them still in the development stage.

Perhaps part of the skepticism surrounding BPD is due to the fact that some of the "traits" inherently associated with having the condition are in themselves, questionable. For example, people with BPD are known to suffer from dissociation. This is an instance when they become detached from emotions and physical experience. As a result, they have a hard time recalling certain events in their past.

This disassociate problem is further compounded by the presumed trait of lying. While there's no conclusive proof that BPD sufferers "lie" as a component of the condition, many people believe that this is one of the symptoms.

In addition, people with BPD are often described as demanding, difficult, manipulative, treatment resistant, violent, and attention seeking. The problem with this negative view that the public has, is it carries the potential for triggering BPD episodes – thereby creating a self-fulfilling prophecy that's hard to get out of. This is why people with BPD often have a problem getting treatment and being taken seriously by the general public.

In the words of Valerie Porr, the president of the Treatment and Research Advancement Association for Personality Disorders, "BPD is …confusing, imparts no relevant or descriptive information, and reinforces existing stigma".

Suggested names to replace BPD include: emotional regulation disorder, emotional dysregulation disorder, interpersonal regulatory disorder, post traumatic personality disorder, and impulse disorder. Unfortunately, none of these have been considered and under the DSM-5 published in the year 2013, the name Borderline Personality Disorder is still used.

Inclusion in Diagnostic and Statistical Manual of Mental Disorders

BPD is also known as Emotionally Unstable Personality Disorder or EUPD. It is officially recognized as a personality disorder under the Diagnostic and Statistical Manual of Mental Disorders. Often, the symptoms of BPD overlap with other mental disorders – such as Bipolar Disorder. For this reason, it's important to obtain a diagnosis from a professional after the professional has considered and eliminated every other possibility.

It was initially introduced in DSM III in 1980 and continues to be part of the Manual. The current edition identifies BPD through 9 diagnostic criteria, where having at least 5 out of the 9 allows for a BPD diagnosis.

Onset of Symptoms

BPD typically occurs during early adulthood but becomes better as a person ages and learns to control and anticipate the symptoms.

Treatment of BPD

Those diagnosed with BPD are considered to be one of the toughest groups to work with during therapy. It requires an excellent skill level in order to successfully engage a BPD sufferer in therapy, and perseverance in gaining positive results from the treatment.

What Causes Borderline Personality Disorder?

The actual cause of BPD is unknown, although genetic factors are noted as the primary possible culprit. Environmental and social factors are also taken into consideration as possible triggers for the onset of symptoms, although the DSM does not view BPD as a stress or trauma related problem. Some cases show that people who have suffered through abuse or neglect as children are more likely to have BPD.

Brain abnormalities are also a likely cause of the problem. Specifically, the portion of the brain dedicated towards impulse control, aggression, and emotion regulation may be damaged – thereby causing BPD symptoms. Any form of trauma or infection that crosses the brain-blood barrier can cause this problem – which means that BPD can result from head injuries, infections, and irregularities in the release and production of brain chemicals.

Risk Factors of BPD
While not everyone who has BPD has had a rough childhood, a problematic young life is one of the risk factors of BPD. Simply put, a child who went through childhood abuse or trauma is more likely to develop BPD as they reach adulthood. It is noted that the 'cause' of BPD often happens during the developmental stage of a person.

If you have a family member who's been diagnosed with Bipolar Personality Disorder or any other personality disorder, then the chances of you developing one yourself in the future are increased.

Types of Borderline Personality Disorder
There are 4 known types of BPD, and treatment is targeted depending on what category your condition falls into.

Discouraged BPD
This type of BPD is characterized by what is primarily codependent and clingy behavior. These are the kind of sufferers who willingly follow the group when making decisions, even though they may not feel 100% into it. This is because they seek approval and will feel absolute dejection if no such approval is forthcoming. They're also the kind that fears abandonment and rejection the most – and are likely to become depressed and self-harming. People who fall under this classification have a sense of anger brimming on the surface for the people around them while at the same time, want attention and approval. Oftentimes, they feel unworthy and unloved.

Impulsive BPD
Impulsive BPD patients can be misleading at first. They're energetic, charismatic, engaging, and may come off as happy extroverts. They seek thrills but can become quickly bored. Impulsives love the attention and excitement of getting into unlikely or abnormal situations. As the name implies, they tend to act first and think about the consequences later. Impulsive types are the ones most likely to seek mind-altering substances such as alcohol and drugs. The need for approval and excitement can also mean engaging in self-harming activities and extravagant activities in order to avoid abandonment and disappointment from loved ones.

Petulant Borderline
A petulant borderline is characterized by symptoms of defiance, impatience, irritability, and unpredictability. They can be quite stubborn and resentful with a pessimistic view of things. Petulants have a sense of unworthiness and are quick to anger. They rely on others but are constantly afraid to end up being disappointed by the same people they rely on. Passive-aggressive traits are common in this type of BPD sufferer, and self-harming is often done to gain attention.

Self-Destructive Borderline
These people are self-loathing and bitter – but rarely realize that they are. They engage in self-destructive behavior but do not see these behaviors as self-destructive, much like an Impulsive. They're terrified of abandonment and will engage in self-harm in order to feel something. Like Impulsives, they're likely to take part in risky behavior such as reckless driving and other dangerous activities.

It's important to note however that an individual may fall within more than one type of BPD classification, depending on the symptoms they manifest. Hence, it's important for therapists to truly observe patients and pay particular attention to the symptoms that lead to their diagnosis. More than anything, it is the accuracy of the therapists' diagnosis and observations that will help create a targeted and effective approach towards treatment.

Sub Categories of People with BPD - Spectrums

It's important to note that over the years, there have been multiple attempts to properly categorize BPD, or to further subdivide it into groups to help target treatment methods. Not all therapists follow these subdivisions, mainly because they're not perfect. Hence, the categorization can be completely subjective, depending on the kind of symptoms you have as identified by a therapist.

In the interest of covering all bases however, this book will still discuss the different categories or divisions of BPD to help you better understand the condition. They are often called "spectrums" because while all three are diagnosed as BPD – the severity of the impact of symptoms may vary from one person to the next.

Low Functioning and Conventional BPDs
These are the patients that people often picture when they think of BPD. The symptoms are fairly obvious, which means that they have a harder time blending in with society. A common sign is if they have a hard time keeping a job or may even be considered disabled due to their mental health. A low functioning Borderline leans toward self-harming and are more likely to contemplate suicide as a coping mechanism. For this reason, they are often hospitalized or listed for inpatient treatment.

Common co-occurring mental health issues for low-functioning Borderline patients include Eating Disorders and Bipolar Personality Disorder. Other determining factors of low functioning Borderlines include:

- They often acknowledge the fact that they have a problem and therefore are more likely to seek treatment, especially if there is encouragement from family and friends.

- Some of them may be on government disability.

- Their overlapping or co-occurring mental health problems are severe enough that they require treatment. In fact, this is often the most obvious thing about them and generally the initial reason why they seek professional help.

- Parents of adolescents with low functioning BPD often fear that their child won't be able to live independently.

- Since low-functioning BPD patients are the ones more likely to seek help, they're also the ones most likely to be part of studies, statistics, and research about the condition.

High Functioning BPD
High functioning Borderlines are also called Invisible Borderline Personalities because they're rarely identified to have the condition. They can function fairly well in society, are often employed and are capable of meeting their responsibilities. They exhibit symptoms of BPD but because of their high functionality, family members and coworkers can become bewildered by their actions. In many cases, they are simply viewed as 'bad' people, especially since their coping techniques can include criticizing others and blaming everyone else but themselves when something goes wrong. Their ability to function in society and hide their main issues means that they will resist or refuse therapy. It doesn't help that a common co-occurring mental health issue for high-functioning BPDs is Narcissistic Personality Disorder.

Other characteristics of those with high functioning BPD include but are not limited to the following:

- They are strongly opposed to any suggestion of mental health problems. In fact, they are of the opinion that issues in work and relationship are because of some other person.

- For this reason, it requires powerful persuasion to get them to see a therapist. Even if they go for counseling, high functioning Borderlines rarely take the therapy seriously.

- The way they deal with pain is outward – that is, they become angry or enraged as opposed to low functioning Borderlines that cope inwards.

- They can function well at work, but their personal relationships are chaotic.

- Some may say that they have a Dr. Jekyll and Mr. Hyde personality as they tend to be aggressive towards those that they are close to.

Combination BPD
As the name suggests, this type falls smack in the middle of the two extremes mentioned above. The main distinction of Combination Borderline patients is the fact that they're willing to obtain help and are often treated as outpatients instead of inpatients. Their coping techniques include anger and rages with a work life that involves frequent disagreements with coworkers. People who fall within the middle spectrum of BPD often have substance abuse and depression as co-occurring mental health issues.

Chapter 2: Symptoms of Borderline Personality Disorder

There are 9 diagnostic symptoms of Borderline Personality Disorder as provided under DSM-IV. Having just 5 of these 9 symptoms is diagnostically read as a confirmation of BPD. Note, however, that a licensed medical professional must make the confirmation.

Fear of Abandonment
While it's perfectly natural for people to fear being left by loved ones, a person with BPD takes it to the extreme. That is, they are afraid of being abandoned and often view even small things as a possible sign of abandonment. For example, a husband can come home late from work, or a parent may go away on a vacation. These are small things but from the perspective of someone with BPD, these instances can trigger intense fear that translates towards negative behavior – such as doing everything you can to keep that person with you. A person with BPD can be quite clingy, requiring a loved one to report often and appraise them of their activities. This can cause a person to move further away instead of bringing them closer.

Unstable Relationships
The diagnostic symptom of unstable relationships for people with BPD usually stems from the unstable swing of emotions. They can fall in love quickly and fall out of love just as quickly. Their relationships are intense at their height and depressing at their lowest – with the full relationships typically being short-lived. There is no in-between for these relationships, as they can be either perfect or horrible, with the switch being rapid and surprising. Family members, friends, and partners may have a hard time keeping up with the swift changes as one bounces from a happy mood to anger, hate, devaluation, and idealization.

Shifting Self Image
Those who suffer from BPD often have an unclear view of themselves. One day, they may love everything about themselves while the next day, they may feel terrible and hate themselves completely. This is why it's not uncommon to find self-harm as a complication of Borderline Personality Disorder. Self-image is just a starting point as sufferers can also feel confused about what they want in life, their values, goals, religion, choice of career, and even choice of friends. Hence, sufferers can change life choices quickly, each time starting a new venture with passion but quickly changing their mind.

Impulsive, Self-Destructive Behavior
Being impulsive every now and then is common for the general population. If you have BPD however, the impulsive behavior is much more prevalent and is done as a sensation-seeking behavior. The impulse is often self-destructive and done when you're experiencing intense emotions such as anger, sadness, anxiety, or depression. The impulse can be spending too much, eating too much, drinking too much, risky sex, reckless driving, or doing drugs.

Self-Harming
Self-harming as a symptom of BPD can be of two types: suicidal or NSSI. The large opinion is that self-harming is indicative of suicidal thoughts or suicidal intention. There could be suicidal threats, gestures, or even actual attempts. NSSI on the other hand is self-harming for the sake of inflicting harm. It is known in the medical community as Non-Suicidal Self Injury, which means that you are only inflicting pain to yourself because you want to experience the feeling. Common self-harm techniques include burning and cutting.

Extreme Emotional Swings
Mood swings for people with BPD are intense but occur in short bursts. You're happy now, sad later, ecstatic the next second, followed by depressed, and then the cycle starts all over again.

The trigger can be small things that are often ignored by other people but can be quite overwhelming for those who have BPD. What makes this distinctive is that people with depression or bipolar disorder often have long lasting mood swings that are present for hours or minutes. People with BPD however, experience this for just a few seconds or a few minutes.

Chronic Feeling of Emptiness

Those with BPD also report a feeling of emptiness that's persistent and chronic. It is described as having a void inside of them – as if they're nothing or no one. For this reason, sufferers may choose to "fill" the void with activities that are viewed as reckless or dangerous. They may choose to do drugs, eat too much, or have indiscriminate sex in order to find something that might be satisfying for them. This rarely helps, however.

Explosive Anger

This is in connection with the rapid change of intense emotions. People with BPD can experience short bursts of intense anger. Sufferers have a very short fuse – which means that it takes very little to set them off. Explosive anger also tends to be physically obvious as sufferers express their anger by throwing things or yelling. There are some instances when the anger is directed inwards however, in which case a sufferer may choose to self-harm or engage in destructive behavior.

Feelings of Suspicion / Out of Touch With Reality

It's also fairly common for people with BPD to be out of touch with reality. This translates to a feeling of suspicion or paranoia about everything that's happening around them. A person with BPD can be suspicious about every little thing, to the point that they can drive people away with their belief of ulterior motives. A sense of detachment can also be present, with sufferers often feeling foggy or out of their own body. There's this spaced out feeling – as if you're watching yourself from a distance.

Disorders That Can Occur Together with BPD

It's important to note that BPD can occur together with other mental health problems such as bipolar disorder or depression. The other mental issues that most often co-occur with BPD include:

- Eating disorders
- Anxiety disorder
- Substance abuse
- Depression
- Bipolar Disorder
- Post-Traumatic Stress Disorder
- Attention Deficit/Hyperactivity Disorder

Should You Trust Online Tests?

No. When it comes to mental health problems, online tests are never a good way of making a firm diagnosis. These can be a good meter when deciding IF you should see a doctor – but it is not a diagnosis in itself.

Borderline Personality Disorder vs. Bipolar Disorder

BPD and Bipolar Disorder are two mental health problems that are often mistaken for each other. It's not really surprising considering how many common symptoms they share. In fact, there are instances when these two conditions can occur at the same time. The precision in diagnosis is important because two different conditions canmean two very different approaches to treatment.

Both conditions involve mood swings and impulsive behavior as symptoms. The key difference however is that BPD is a mood disorder while BPD is a personality disorder. Mood disorders are characterized primarily by serious mood swings, while Personality disorders are linked towards how a person thinks or feels.

Borderline Personality Disorder vs Antisocial Personality Disorder

These two conditions have many overlapping symptoms including disinhibition, impulsiveness, and self-harming tendencies. In fact, both conditions fall within the Cluster B Classification in the DSM-5 which is characterized by a dramatic, overly emotional, and unpredictable manner of thinking and behavior. Certain distinctions however can be noted, specifically with the degree of emotions considered. Those with ASPD have few emotions while people with BPD have extreme emotions of varying types. The treatment for these two conditions is also very different, thereby requiring an accurate diagnosis.

Chapter 3: Diagnosis of Borderline Personality Disorder

Due to the complexity of the condition, diagnosing BPD can be a challenge. While the DSM has set up a concrete list of diagnostic criteria for health professionals – it's still necessary to dig deep and fully understand the patient before making a definitive diagnosis. In making a diagnosis therefore, it's important to look at different aspects of the condition. Here's how a typical diagnosis process for BPD proceeds:

- Detailed interview with a mental health provider
- Psychological evaluation including answering questionnaires
- Medical history and exam
- Discussion of signs and symptoms

Diagnosis in Age Groups
A diagnosis of BPD is rarely made in children. Typically, it is the adults who are affirmatively diagnosed with BPD. Symptoms of BPD in children are often associated with other mental health problems. This is because BPD symptoms can disappear in children as they mature.

Brain Scans for Diagnosis
As mentioned in the previous Chapter, there are marked differences between the brain of a person with BPD and those who do not have the condition. Note though that as of this writing, brain scans are used to aid BPD diagnosis – but it's not the conclusive diagnostic method. It's likely that brain scans will play a bigger role in future diagnosis of BPD as well as possible treatments for the condition. As of now however, it is used only in conjunction with other diagnostic methods.

Mental Health Professionals
Note that diagnosing BPD is best done by a specialist such as a psychiatrist or a psychologist. An initial appointment is often done with your primary care physician who will then direct you to a mental health provider.

Preparing for an Initial Appointment
During your initial appointment, your doctor or the mental health professional will ask questions to determine the existence of a mental health condition. At the initial stages of the diagnosis, the mental health professional shall first consider all the possibilities – so the questions will be generalized. Even if *you* think you have Borderline Personality Disorder, a good physician will consider all the possibilities and eliminate them one by one, as symptoms indicate.

Common questions that will be asked include:

- Any symptoms you've noticed, how often they occur, and how long they are present.

- Medical information such as physical health and mental health problems you've had in the past.

- Traumatic events in your past as well as present stressors in your life.

- All medications you have taken in the past or are currently taking.

- How the symptoms are affecting your life, specifically in terms of work relationships, family life, and romantic relationships.

- How well you manage the intense emotions and mood swings.

- How often do you feel abandoned or victimized.

- How do you describe your sense of self-worth.

- If you've ever had instances of self-destructive, impulsive, or risky behavior.

- How often you drink, smoke, or use prescription drugs for recreation.

- A description of your childhood, including your relationship with parents and guardians.

- Patient history – specifically if any of your relatives have been diagnosed with mental health problems.

Take a Friend or Family Member
It's usually a good idea to have a friend or family member with you when meeting a mental health professional. This has to be a person you trust and who has watched you during the emergence of these symptoms. Input from a close friend or family member will make it easier for a health professional to properly label the symptoms and make the correct conclusions.

Ask Questions
Finally, don't hesitate to ask questions of the medical professional. Depending on the stage of the diagnosis, the doctor may not be able to give a definitive diagnosis of the condition, but should be able to give a list of possibilities – based on the information you've given them.

How Long Does Diagnosis Usually Take?
Diagnosis usually occurs right after the assessment, but this may vary from one professional to the next. The assessment itself can take some time, often covering a full day with the physician. It is only after they've gone through every single result will they be comfortable in making a diagnosis. In some

cases, they may even refer you for further testing, or to another professional. The fact is that BPD, like many other mental health conditions, is an inexact science. There are many overlapping conditions and studies that constantly impose changes on how the condition is viewed. This being the case, health care professionals are very careful before making a diagnosis.

Chapter 4: Brain Function of a Person with BPD

Thanks to new medical technology such as MRIs (Magnetic Resonance Imaging), the brains of people with BPD have been studied to see if there are structural problems or any difference in how their brains function. The results of the study have been illuminating as doctors note certain aspects of the brain that correspond with the known symptoms of BPD.

Amygdala
To start with, people with BPD have a smaller amygdala. This is the part of the brain which regulates fear and aggression. Also known as the "primitive part of the brain", people with BPD have a more hyperactive amygdala, which means that they can experience emotions more intensely. This also means that it takes them longer to recover from an intense emotion.

Hippocampus
There's also a difference with how the hippocampus reacts for people with BPD. This part of the brain is basically the emotional reaction decider of the body. It accepts external data, processes it, and decides on the proper emotional response for what just happened. It can choose to approach the problem or avoid it, basically a "fight or flight" decision. People with BPD have their hippocampus constantly aroused. This means that they're always in this "alert" state of mind to the point where even non-threats are perceived as threats. The hippocampus then relays this misdiagnosis to the amygdala, which then generates the response.

Prefrontal Cortex
The prefrontal cortex is the part of the brain that really separates humans from the rest of the beings in the Kingdom of Animalia. It is what defines human evolution as the prefrontal cortex is responsible for rationality and logic in connection with

decision-making. It battles with the primal nature of humans, allowing them to make decisions based on reason. While people with BPD still have a prefrontal cortex, it is underperforming. Hence, they have the symptom of impulsiveness as noted under the DSM.

Insula

Next, we have the brain area called the insula which is primarily responsible for how a person experiences negative emotions. It is mainly concerned with the intensity of negative emotions felt. For a person with BPD, the insula is hyperactive, which means that negative emotions have a higher impact on them. While some people can easily brush off certain negative emotions, these feelings for them linger and are harder to deal with. Combine this with the fact that they have less 'brakes" or ability to put a stop to those negative thoughts, and you get one of the major diagnostic symptoms of BPD.

Hypothalamic Pituitary Adrenal Axis

This is the name given for 3 interconnected glands – the hypothalamus, the pituitary, and the adrenal gland. When interacting with each other, these three are capable of regulating how a person perceives and handles pressure. They're also the main parts that control cortisol production – also known as the stress regulating hormone. People with BPD have irregular activity in these glands. This means that they produce more cortisol levels than they're supposed to – thereby causing the body to feel more stressed, even during non-stressful moments.

Brain Chemicals Involved

After talking about the various parts of the brain involved, the next step is to look closer at the brain chemicals involved in BPD. So far, 3 have been closely looked into by researchers, and this is what they have found:

- Opiates – ordinarily, opiates are released by the body to increase pain tolerance. It helps dull the pain as a response to tissue damage. Hence, the more opiates you have in your body, the higher your level of pain tolerance. Accordingly, people with BPD resorting to self-harm have lower amounts of opiates in their body. This means that although they may not be aware of it, people with BPD self-harm in order to naturally increase the opiates in their body – thus making them able to tolerate pain.

- Serotonin – serotonin is primarily concerned with the regulation of sleep, learning, and moods. According to studies, people with BPD have low levels of serotonin in their body. Low levels are associated with suicide, anxiety, depression, and appetite regulation. In some cases, impulsive aggression is also connected with low levels of serotonin.

- Cortisol – finally, we have cortisol which is popularly known as a stress hormone. Cortisol actually has benefits in that it can help with the breakdown of proteins and carbohydrates. Just the right amount of it in the body can therefore help convert sugar into energy. The problem is when you have too much of it. If present for long periods of time, it can cause an unhealthy buildup of fat, increase blood pressure, as well as sugar levels in the body. It can also impact immune system function, leading to sped up aging. There's also a negative impact on the brain's memory center.

What Does This Mean for Treatment?
So, if there are structural and functional brain problems for people with BPD – does this mean that there's no hope towards solving this mental health problem? Of course not.

Studies have shown that there are techniques and methods that can help an individual better train his or her thinking process so that more emphasis is put on reason and logic, and less emphasis on impulsiveness. Some exercises that will be discussed in this book also implement methods that help improve brain matter – thereby causing better impulse control for people with BPD. Just because there are brain-level issues affecting how a person with BPD functions, it doesn't mean there's no treatment available.

Mental health issues are definitely among the aspects of health that are currently getting lots of attention. As of the writing of this book, there are still more developments and research being conducted to help people with BPD cope better in their day to day life.

Chapter 5: What Happens During a BPD Episode

If you go online, you'll find that there are lots of videos showing how a Borderline Personality Disorder episode occurs. Chances are that these images are already familiar to you – but have you ever tried to break down what you're feeling from the moment the anxiety sets in, the emotion climaxes, and the eventual ebb of the emotion?

A BPD Episode can be segmented into steps, and therapists can label these steps differently. Usually though, it is composed of just 3 major segments. These are: (1) the trigger; (2) the climax; and (3) the aftermath.

Understanding the Trigger

The "trigger" is the event that gets the ball rolling. It is the activity that causes the emergence of the episode. Now, the trigger may vary from one person to the next – which means that the trigger for one patient may not be the same for another. It's also important to note that triggers can be completely mundane things. People without BPD can experience the same events without any issue, but for someone with BPD, the event is something that can cause deep anxiety.

Triggers can be classified into two things: external or internal.

An external trigger is something that occurs outside your mind. It could happen to you or it could be something you witnessed. An internal trigger is something that occurs primarily in your mind. It's an assumption, a memory, or a thought that makes you go off the deep end.

Now, there are different types of triggers today as discussed below:

Relationship Triggers
This is perhaps the most common type of BPD trigger. Relationships here are taken to mean all types of relationships from family, work, or romantic. Events that make a person feel abandoned or rejected can easily create impulsive behaviors, self-harm, and depression. It can be something as intense as a fight with a partner, or as abstract as a friend who fails to call back after promising to make the call. For some people, a friend who forgets to call is a negligible problem – but for someone with BPD, it can lead to extreme deductions. Sufferers may think that their friend just didn't want to talk to them or that this friend doesn't really like them or is mad at them. You'll notice that this trigger is a combination of the two classifications: the external and the internal. Externally, a friend fails to do something and internally, the BPD patient starts to assume scenarios that generate the symptoms.

Cognitive Triggers
Cognitive triggers are completely internal and can occur completely out of thin air. These are often in the form of a flashback or a memory such as past abuse or past trauma. A loss of a loved one is also a possible trigger. Some BPD sufferers report that even a good memory can trigger the trauma. Specifically, it can cause a person to compare the past and the present, arriving at a conclusion that their life right now is nowhere as good as it was before.

The Climax
The climax of a BPD episode is characterized as the part where an individual loses control. You've failed to manage the trigger, and now will begin to experience the intense emotions. You're furious, depressed, anxious, or even feeling incredibly impulsive. Some Borderline persons describe it as a feeling like

a primal animal where all that matters is your survival. Therefore, you're in a fight or flight mode and you seem to be stuck on that feeling of perpetual doom.

The emotion is so strong that there's practically nothing a person can do or say to jolt you out of that emotional rollercoaster. Verbally, you may be yelling or cursing at people. Physically, you may be hurting them or perhaps you're crying and contemplating suicidal thoughts. Physical manifestations of fear such as shaking, shouting, crying, and goosebumps are quite common as well. Some BPD sufferers also report having both auditory and visual hallucinations during their worst episodes. Disassociation is also likely during this time with individuals going completely mute and unresponsive.

So, what can be done during this time? Grounding exercises can help, but this requires that you be able to recognize that you're in the middle of an episode. Most BPD sufferers ride it out – which means that they suffer through the moment – because they have no other choice. However, you'll find during therapy that this doesn't always have to be the case. There are techniques that can help stop the climax or at least, keep it as short as possible. Having external sources of help – such as a family member or a friend – can also help with the recovery after climax.

The Aftermath
The Aftermath is when things go back to zero. At this point, you feel utterly exhausted, calm, and numb – all at the same time. It has been described as if you're a blank slate and all the negative emotions have been cried out. It's a moment of complete mental silence and for many, it feels like complete relief.

How Long Does an Episode Last?
A full BPD episode can last for hours, depending on the stage in which a person is in their treatment. The problem however is that an episode rarely happens in the singular. BPD is a cycle,

which means that there can be multiple episodes within a single day.
Hence, after the aftermath, you get a few hours of respite before symptoms may come back. Oftentimes, Borderlines remember the trigger and the cycle starts all over again.

What Happens After the Cycle?
So, let's say you've had 3 Episodes and the cycle is over. What happens next? Unfortunately, the next plethora of emotions has nothing to do with BPD but has everything to do with how you feel about having BPD. Simply put, you might feel guilty, regretful, remorseful, anxious, or self-loathing after a BPD Cycle. These emotions will come charging into your mind after a Cycle as a natural response to what happened.

At this stage, you become completely aware of the fact that you just went through a BPD Cycle. Some thoughts that may be rushing in to your consciousness include:

Why am I like this?
I should have managed the trigger.
I should have been able to stop at the trigger.
I should have managed during the Climax.
I hate myself.
I'm too stupid to use the treatment.
I'll never recover from this.
I'll never have a normal life.
I'll never be able to manage this.

Have a Record of an Episode
It also helps to take a video of yourself during an episode, or perhaps an audio recording, or just have someone recount to you what happened during the moment. It also helps to have an external perspective of what occurred during the episode since many BP persons tend to focus only internally so much that they lose track of their actions. Keep a video of it, record it, or if it happened while with a friend, have them tell you exactly what you did, how you acted, and their perception of what happened. This will give you a better idea on what you do during an

episode and therefore, what you *can* do in order to curb the negative actions.

Chapter 6: Treatments for Borderline Personality Disorder

So how exactly is BPD treated? There are actually several methods for treatment. However, before we discuss all of those, we should first look into the different mental health professionals who can accurately make the diagnosis and recommend treatment.

Mental Health Professionals

There are multiple mental health professionals today, categorized depending on the kind of services they provide and to whom. If you or a loved one is suspected to have BPD, it's usually a good idea to seek help from your primary physician before going to a mental health professional.

The following mental health professionals are capable of providing therapy and psychological assessments. However, they generally cannot issue prescriptions, with some exceptions in certain States.

Clinical Psychologist

This is a person who has a doctoral degree in psychology from an accredited program. They have the power to make diagnoses and conduct both individual and group therapy. In conjunction, there's also the School Psychologist who is capable of performing the same things, but primarily functions within a school and works well with school staff to maximize the efficiency of a campus in addressing mental health problems.

Clinical Social Worker

Often found in hospitals, a clinical social worker is someone who has a master's degree in social work and are trained to make diagnoses of mental health conditions. They're also capable of conducting treatment through individual and group counseling.

Mental Health Counselor

A counselor is someone who has a master's degree and supervised clinical work experience. They can diagnose and provide counseling.

Pastoral Counselor

This is someone who has clinical pastoral education and is capable of diagnosing and providing counseling. They're part of the clergy and are a good choice for patients who have a strong religious background and want to use this to help them through recovery.

Licensed Professional Counselor

This is someone who has a master's degree in psychology and counseling. They can offer diagnoses and conduct counseling, either in a group, or individually.

Nurse Psychotherapist

While capable of conducting counseling, this practitioner has the status of a registered nurse who went through specialized training for mental health nursing.

Certified Alcohol and Drug Abuse Counselor

This type of counselor is ideal for those whose BPD symptoms are manifested through substance abuse. They can target and treat the complications more readily, often through counseling.

Peer Specialist

This is a type of counselor who has personal experience with mental health problems and can therefore approach the topic from a relatable perspective. They've also gone through training and can therefore assists clients with respect to recovery by teaching them how to develop and achieve goals.

Marital and Family Therapist

These are ideal for households that want to help a member work through their mental health issues. A family therapist has a master's degree and special education catering towards this specific niche. They can provide counseling individually or as part of a group.

On the other hand, the following professionals can prescribe medications but cannot conduct therapy:

Psychiatrist

A psychiatrist is a medical doctor having special training with the treatment of mental and emotional health problems. There are different types of psychiatrists that include a child/adolescent psychiatrist and a mental health nurse practitioner. A child psychiatrist, as the name implies, is one who primarily caters to children.

Mental Health Nurse Practitioner

Registered nurse practitioners can also provide treatment and diagnosis of mental health problems, provided they've had a graduate degree and specialized training in the field.

Other Therapists

Some therapists also specialize in certain fields, depending on what aspects the patient responds to best. For example, some patients may love music in which case, there are music therapists who can use this music as a medium to help their patients.

Treating BPD with Psychotherapy

Psychotherapy is the most common manner in which BPD is treated. Note though that it may be administered together with specific medications. Psychotherapy also goes by the term "talk therapy" and comes in many types.

Dialectical Behavior Therapy

Also known as DBT, this method makes use of both individual and group approaches to treat Borderline Personality Disorder. It encourages the development of certain skills that can help with the management of emotions as they arise. Using this therapy method, you can also develop techniques in order to better handle distress and relationship with other people.

Mentalization Based Therapy

Through this therapy, you can learn how to identify your own thoughts and feelings within a given moment. With identification, you can move on towards understanding and further, towards the generation of alternative perspectives relative to the situation. With MBT, you are taught how to think about a situation and analyze it completely before reacting accordingly. It essentially forces you to use the prefrontal cortex more actively so that reasoning and logic is properly utilized.

Schema Focused Therapy

This particular method of treating BPD puts the focus on unmet needs that caused the creation of negative habits in life. The goal is to identify those needs and find a way to meet them in a healthy manner so that you do not resort to negative habits. This manner of talk therapy can be approached either individually or as a group.

Systems Training for Emotional Predictability and Problem Solving

This is a 20-week treatment method that primarily focuses on group work. Also known as STEPSS, it encourages the participation of family members, friends, significant others, and caregivers in the treatment. Note though that this is a course of action that's usually taken together with other methods of psychotherapy.

Transference Focused Psychotherapy

This method helps patients understand their emotions and other difficulties on an interpersonal level. A trust relationship is encouraged between you and your therapist to help develop insights into your own personality. This insight is then applied to all ongoing situations, leaving you a little bit better with handling relationships.

Good Psychiatric Management

This method is anchored primarily on case management. It involves school and work participation where patients are encouraged to make full sense of their emotional difficulties. They are asked to analyze their emotionally difficult moments and consider interpersonal causations for these feelings. This therapy technique often includes family education, group input, medication, and individual therapy.

Despite the varying classes of psychotherapy however, all types consider the following:

- Your current ability to function
- How you manage your emotions
- Your understanding of the scope and gravity of your symptoms
- How to reduce your impulsiveness
- How to become aware of your feelings and how to handle them
- Work towards improving relationships with other people
- Understand more about borderline personality disorder

Dialectical Behavior Therapy
Abbreviated to DBT, this is a type of cognitive behavioral therapy popular as treatment for those who have Borderline Personality Disorder. DBT works by targeting negative behaviors in people diagnosed with mental health problems. These negative behaviors are eliminated by teaching brand new behaviors to replace the bad ones. It's a 4-step approach that includes the following:

- Mindfulness
- Distress tolerance
- Interpersonal effectiveness
- Emotion regulation

There are two sets of skills introduced and taught through DBT. These are the What Skills and the How Skills.

The What Skills help the client learn the following:
- Observe their day to day experience
- Be able to describe their experience through verbal labels
- Become fully present in the moment and be aware of their actions without being self-conscious

The How Skills are more focused outwards, teaching patients how to observe and interact with their experiences. Here are the typical components of How Skills:

- Learn to go through experiences in a non-judgmental or non-evaluative manner
- Learn to focus on just one thing at a time, as well as realign their thoughts or bring back their attention if it starts to wander
- Keep their focus on their goals regardless of their mood

Treating BPD with Medication

It is important to note that there is no specific medication being used for BPD. As of this writing, no drug has been approved by the Food and Drug Administration with respect to Borderline Personality Disorder. Some drugs, however, can be prescribed to help with the symptoms or complications associated with the condition. For example, there are drugs used for depression, anxiety, and aggression.

The following are some of the most common medications being used today:

Antidepressants

This includes the use of SSRIs or selective serotonin reuptake inhibitors. They're the first line of defense when it comes to addressing depressive episodes. As the name suggests, they were originally made for people suffering from major depressive disorders. Since depression is often a co-occurring condition of BPD, it's also not surprising that antidepressants are prescribed if it becomes necessary. When taken, the medication can help with low mood, anxiety, sadness, and emotional reactivity. Common antidepressants include:

- Nardil (phenelzine)
- Effexor (venlafaxine)
- Wellbutrin (bupropion)
- Prozac (fluoxetine)
- Zoloft (sertraline)

Antipsychotics

This includes Zyprexa which can help reduce hostility, impulsivity, and psychotic symptoms associated with BPD. One thing you should know is that "borderline" was originally coined as such because according to medical professionals, BPD symptoms were on the border of psychosis and neurosis. This is why antipsychotics were originally used to treat BPD and fortunately, studies show that they actually have a positive effect on sufferers of the condition. When taken correctly, they can help reduce paranoid thinking, hostility, anxiety, and impulsiveness of patients.

Common antipsychotics taken include but are not limited to the following:

- Haldol (haloperidol)
- Zyprexa (olanzapine)
- Clozaril (clozapine)
- Seroquel (quetiapine)
- Risperdal (risperidone) (Risperdal)

Anti-Anxiety Medications

Common drugs include Xanax, Valium, Ativan, and Klonopin. Anxiety is a common co-occurring condition with BPD, which is why those with the condition are often prescribed anti-anxiety drugs. Notably however, there's very little research to support the use of anti-anxiety medicines for people with BPD. In fact, some medications can worsen BPD symptoms – specifically Ativan and Klonopin. Make sure to discuss this with your physician before choosing to take any of the prescribed medications falling under this category. Also note that BPD patients suffering some substance abuse may find these medications to be habit forming.

Here's a list of common anti-anxiety medications:

- Ativan (lorazepam)
- Klonopin (clonazepam)
- Xanax (alprazolam)
- Valium (diazepam)
- Buspar (buspirone)

Mood Stabilizers

This includes Topamax, Depakote, and Lamictal, all of which are good in treating aggression from BPD. They work not just as mood stabilizers but also as anticonvulsants. In BPD patients, they can help with impulsive behavior as well as regulate rapid changes in emotion. Here are some of the common medications under this category:

- Lithobid (lithium carbonate)
- Depakote (valproate)
- Lamictal (lamotrigine)
- Tegretol or Carbatrol (carbamazepine)

Choosing Proper BPD Medication

While you might think that choosing BPD medication is completely up to your physician, this is not entirely the case. The fact is that your current needs and health status are taken into consideration when your physician decides on the proper BPD medication to use. What you should understand is that there is no single drug for BPD. Prescription will cover several drugs types – a veritable cocktail that's designed to target different symptoms of the condition.

When discussing what is the best medication to take, be upfront about your needs and the side-effects you want to avoid. In many cases, medication will be adjusted depending on how you react to it. Through different sessions, your physician will ask how you're faring with the current medication and make adjustments as needed.

CBD as Treatment for BPD

CBD is a product of marijuana, but without the intoxicating effect. Although it is still currently a hot topic for politicians today, the use of CBD now less stringent limitations. For one thing, CBD is now legal in certain doses. It can also be bought in different forms such as CBD oil, CBD chocolate, and other CBD-infused products.

But what can it do for people with CBD? CBD is often associated with medical marijuana, which is currently being used for numerous health problems. Accordingly, CBD can help reduce anxiety and increase pain tolerance. While CBD is a treatment that won't be immediately be considered by your physician, it at least deserves to be asked about – just in case the treatment would be a more welcome alternative. Note that CBD as treatment for BPD is still untested and has not been properly confirmed. Given the legal limitations, not all mental health professionals will feel confident prescribing it to their patients.

Recommending Hospitalization

Hospitalization may be recommended for individuals who experience self-harm or may be a harm to others. It may also be needed for those who need intense medical treatment or monitoring in order to guarantee that all medications and therapeutic necessities are being met.

How Treatment Will Help

Treatment of BPD does not cure or eradicate the symptoms of the condition. However, it does provide the patient with a better grasp of their emotions. Impulse control is heightened so that you'll have a better handle on how you respond to certain triggers. It can also help control co-occurring problems such as substance abuse, depression, or self-harming.

How Long Does Treatment Take?

Treatment can take anywhere from months to years – depending on the severity of the symptoms. This is because patients are taught how to manage their emotions, thoughts, and behavior – all of which takes time and patience. There are steps that must be taken, and the goal is to turn them into deeply ingrained habits that patients can use each time they feel overwhelmed with emotions.

The symptoms therefore are always present. You will always struggle with the symptoms of BPD – but your response to these symptoms will vary greatly through successful treatment. Over time, your ability to function becomes better so that you'll feel good not just about yourself but the general world around you.

In some cases, treatment never really stops. Visits to a therapist persist but only become slightly farther apart as you get better at handling the symptoms.

Chapter 7: Finding the Right Therapist

Having the right therapist is incredibly influential in how a person with BPD progresses in their management of symptoms. This is why it's very important for you to look for a therapist that you are comfortable with, and you can trust to steer you in the right direction. While the process of finding one can be confusing, frustrating, and time consuming – you will note that choosing the right person will provide great leaps towards recovery. In contrast, the "wrong" psychotherapist won't really help you advance but instead, foster regression and worsen symptoms of BPD.

With that being the case, here's what you should take note of when looking for a BPD therapist or counselor:

Your Current Location
How far are you willing to travel in order to visit your therapist? You might also want to consider the kind of transportation you'll be using to and from your preferred therapist, as well as your preferred schedule for visits. Make a point of listing all of these things down so you can easily talk through it when meeting with someone for the first time.

Once you've considered the location that you're willing to find a therapist in, lock that down and do a Google search. It's usually a good idea to ask your primary care physician for an initial recommendation, but the opposite is also possible. You can narrow down your choices first and ask your primary care physician for their input on the people you've listed.

Insurance Coverage
You're going to consider cost twice when looking for a qualified therapist. The first is before you find one and the second is when you're actually talking with your therapist. If you perform an insurance check at first, then you'll feel confident about

walking into any mental health office, knowing that your initial session is covered.

Call your insurance provider and ask them about your health insurance, specifically the coverage with respect to mental health needs. You'll want to know how they treat visits to the therapist, and how many sessions are covered. Some insurance providers only accommodate health sessions when done with therapists accredited under their system.

Also note that some therapists only accept out-of-pocket payments. This means that they will issue a receipt that you can show to your insurance provider for reimbursement.

Your Current Needs
It's also important to do a self-evaluation as to where you are in your BPD diagnosis. There are several stages to consider:

- First, you're only looking for an evaluation of a mental health problem. In this case, there is no diagnosis yet. A full assessment is necessary before a more targeted approach towards finding a therapist can begin. This being the case, you can go to any mental health professional to create a treatment plan.

- If you've already been diagnosed and are only looking for a psychotherapist, decide whether you need someone long-term or short-term. If you're seeking short-term treatment, then chances are you want to address a specific issue related to BPD.

- If you're in a crisis however, it's best to seek emergency help. Call family members, friends, or the hotline in your location for immediate help. If you're inclined towards self-harming or harming someone else, then this is the best way to deal with the condition at hand.

Type and Level of Expertise
An assessment will give you an idea of what kind of therapist you're looking for. For example, if your main problem is with alcohol abuse, then you can find someone who specializes in that specific field of BPD sufferers. Note that a high level of expertise can also mean high costs per session.

Therapist Orientation
Therapy is inexact science and while progress has been documented, there are still varying schools of thought with respect to how psychotherapy is approached. Different therapists coming from different places may therefore subscribe to different schools of thought when approaching BPD.

Here are the different schools of thought when it comes to psychotherapy:

Humanistic Psychotherapy
This is a client-centered approach to therapy with the intent of creating optimal conditions for the personal growth of the patient. It takes into consideration all aspects of human experience, specifically the day to day experience of the patient. Through this method, the therapist shall make use of the individual's experience as a jump-off point for creating therapeutic goals through step-by-step self-learning activities. The most distinctive aspect of Humanistic Psychotherapy is the engenderment of self-responsibility and reinforcing self-empowerment.

Person Centered Therapy
Another client-centered manner of therapy, this technique focuses on showing empathy, openness, and positivity towards the client. Developed by Carl Rogers in the 1940s, the underlying theory under this therapy is that every person has the capacity to fulfill his own potential and will happily strive towards reaching it. The goal of the therapist therefore is to

create an environment that fosters this natural human potential through empathy and unconditional positive regard. The therapist is there to support, guide, and help to create a structure towards treatment. Through this school of thought, the therapist-client connection must be genuine so that the client can open up and show vulnerability.

Expressive Therapy

This is any form of therapy that makes use of artistic expression as a way of treating patients. They use different disciplines of the creative arts including drawing, dancing, drama, music, and writing. The core belief of this approach is that clients are best treated through an expression of their imagination, while at the same time through integrating the issues in their day to day life with the intent of creating a solution.

Systemic

This therapy approach takes into consideration the input of the group towards the wellbeing of the patient as opposed to an individual approach. Most therapies target the individual, but the systemic approach promotes family therapy and marriage counseling. It also takes into consideration community psychology, whereupon small groups are used to help with the management of personality disorders. Nowadays, group therapy is fairly common and may be integrated alongside other therapy approaches.

Cognitive Behavioral Therapy

Also known as CBT, this approach is perhaps one of the most popular talk therapy techniques being used today. It is a structured method that encourages the patient to recognize and become aware of negative thinking, followed by steps to prevent it from overtaking a person's mind. Through CBT, individuals can learn how to properly respond to BPD episodes so that they'll achieve a fairly normal day-to-day life. When combined with other therapy types, CBT is found to be incredibly helpful in treating all forms of mental health problems.

Gestalt Therapy
The Gestalt therapy approach to psychotherapy is client-centered. This helps clients focus on the present and understand what is really happening in their lives right now, rather than what they may perceive is happening based on their past experience. Instead of just talking about past situations, the client is encouraged to experience them, perhaps through re-enactment. Through the gestalt process, clients learn to become more aware of how their own negative thought patterns and behaviors are blocking true self-awareness and are making them unhappy.

Insight Oriented Therapy

Insight-oriented psychotherapy is a traditional "talk" therapy that delves into how life events, desires, past and current relationships, and unconscious conflicts affect your feelings and contribute to your anxiety. During your treatment, you and your therapist identify compromises you've made to defend yourself against painful thoughts or emotions, and examine how they relate to your current distress.

While the duration of insight-oriented therapy can be open-ended, a variation called brief dynamic therapy that is limited to a specific period (generally 12 to 20 weeks) is often used to target generalized anxiety.

Post-Modernist Therapy

Child Psychotherapy
This method of psychotherapy is specially formulated to meet the needs of children. Considering the difference in the mental development of kids, a unique approach has to be created to meet their specific needs. Note though that therapists are usually reluctant to make a BPD diagnosis with children – which is why the therapy rarely focuses on a BPD condition, and instead merely addresses the likely causes of these symptoms.

Computer Supported Psychotherapy
This one is fairly new but is growing in popularity as computers become a staple in daily life. Applications such as virtual reality or computer-generated scenarios are being introduced in the field of psychology to help patients immerse themselves in experiences and formulate healthy responses in the given setting. It's possibly one of the best ways to teach self-help strategies, such as grounding exercises.

Other computer-supported therapy techniques include tele-therapy or the use of modern communication devices such as videos, texts, and emails. This can be helpful for patients who need someone to talk to during an impending episode.

Questions to Ask the Therapist

- Are you a state-licensed psychologist?
- Is your license active?
- Where did you get your degree?
- How long have you been taking clients?
- What is your area of expertise?
- What kind of training or clinical experience have you had with my kind of problem?
- What kind of treatment do you use?
- How effective is the treatment when dealing with my kind of situation?
- How can you tell if the treatment is working?
- How long will treatment last?
- How much do you charge, and do you accept insurance?
- What is your availability? When is the earliest appointment you can schedule for me?
- Do you see people for long-term or short-term therapy? How long are the sessions?
- What is your approach for my problem?
- What is your goal for this therapy?
- What level of participation do you need from me?
- How long have you been practicing?

- What certification and licenses do you have?
- What professional organization do you belong to?
- How much do you charge?
- When was the last time you worked with someone having the same condition as me?
- How many clients have you had that have the same problem as me?
- How are those clients? Are you still seeing them?
- Describe your ideal patient.
- How do you approach treatment? Do you primarily guide your patients or are you more directive?
- How often do you consult with peers?
- How often do you think you'll see me and for how long?
- How do you set up goals for treatment? What is success for you? How do we know we're there?
- What are the sessions like and how long are they?
- What kind of homework do you give patients?
- How will I prepare for my first session?

Questions to Ask Yourself After Seeing a Therapist

- Do you feel as though the therapist listened to your problems?
- Do you feel respected by the therapist?
- Was the therapist condescending?
- Did the therapist seem like he's just playing a role?
- Was the therapist passive or active during the session? Do you like this method of interaction?
- Did you feel worse or better after the session?
- Did you feel comfortable with the therapist?
- Did you feel safe during the session?

Seek Referrals

Finally, don't forget to ask around about the quality of the therapist. While you can ask for referrals from family, friends, and your primary care physician – the fact is that they may not always come up to scratch. For this reason, you can look up online resources to find a good therapist or at least find out more about your narrowed down choices. Some good online sources include the Ucompare Healthcare Psychiatrist Search, the American Psychological Association, and the Association for Behavioral and Cognitive Therapies.

Chapter 8: Lifestyle Treatment Methods

Alternative treatment methods can be classified into two types: immediate and lifestyle. It's important to use *both* treatment methods, and not just one as they will complement each other as you move through life.

As the name implies, an immediate alternative treatment is something that will best help you during an episode. Some examples include Grounding Exercises or Outlet Exercises which are discussed in a later chapter.

Lifestyle alternative treatments however are those methods that are incorporated in your daily life such as meditation, eating properly, and exercising. In this chapter, we'll be focusing on the Lifestyle Alternative Treatment methods. By incorporating these methods into your life, you will find it easier to identify looming episodes, minimize the occurrences of these episodes, stop an episode from progressing, properly handle a climax, and learn how to make yourself feel better during the aftermath.

Keep a Mood Diary
It can be argued that a Mood Diary falls within the definition of an Outlet, and that's completely true. However, a mood diary also helps you to identify patterns in your BPD episodes. While it might seem like your episodes happen completely at random, the fact is that your triggers are more or less similar in nature.

After a BPD cycle – go back and think about what happened that triggered the episode. Write that down. What happened before the episode? What did you feel? How long did the episode last? How were you able to end the cycle? What techniques did you use to help you manage the emotional roller coaster?

Be as specific as possible in your mood diary, writing down not just the particulars of the event but also the time, the place, the day, how the rest of your day went, the food you ate, and even what you did and felt hours before the episode occurred.

By documenting all this information, you'll find that there is a pattern to these events. There are things you *do* that may trigger these episodes, or perhaps there are people you *meet* that make it tough for you to handle your emotions. It can be something completely random or it can be something that makes sense, but that you've failed to notice until now.

It's also important to take note of things when they're going well. What were you doing that made you feel good?

Managing Your Triggers
In this chapter, we'll talk about how to manage triggers in order to help you with a BPD episode. Typically, the best approach is to avoid the trigger altogether. This means that when you know that *something* can cause you to undergo an episode, make the smart decision to walk away from the confrontation.

Learn the Distinction between BPD and the Complications
Complications associated with BPD are often viewed as a single thing, instead of being associated with BPD itself. This usually occurs when the BPD is undiagnosed or when the patient is a high functioning BPD sufferer. For example, alcohol abuse can occur in people with BPD. They can also have relationship problems, engage in risky behavior and lose jobs regularly. It's important to consider the likelihood that these people suffer from substance abuse BECAUSE of BPD instead of thinking that they have BPD *and* substance abuse.

Build a Support System
Creating a support system can go a long way in helping you through the day to day trials of BPD. Your support system can be composed of different people – your friends, family members, an understanding coworker, a good boss, a teacher, a

fellow student, or other people who have BPD. Note though that you can only forge a great support system by being upfront about the problem in the first place. You need to be honest about your situation and what you need so that in turn, people will be honest with you. This requires a delicate balance that can be tough and in itself, can create pressure for people with BPD. However, your therapist should be able to help and provide you with the assistance and support-building skills that you need.

Food Products that Can Help

Now, there is no definitive list of food or dietary items that have been proven to treat BPD – at least, not as it stands alone. This means that while there are food items you can take to help with BPD symptoms, they're usually taken together with medications and therapy.

Here are some of the dietary additions that can help boost your treatment plans:

Omega 3 Fatty Acids
Research done by Doctors Mary Zanarini and Frances Frankenburg showed that supplementing your diet with 1000 mg of omega-3 fatty acids could help decrease episodes of aggression and depression in patients. The study was done during a course of 8 weeks on both adults and adolescents with BPD. This was done after it was noted that people with mental health problems are deficient in omega-3 fatty acids. This isn't just true for BPD patients but also for those diagnosed with bipolar disorder, schizophrenia, ADHD, and depression.

Fortunately, omega-3 fatty acids are readily available in capsule and gel form as supplements. You can also consume them from food items like cold water fish, walnuts, Brussels sprouts, flax seed, cauliflower hemp seed, hemp oil, and grass-fed beef. Note that your consumption should be limited to the amount prescribed on the label or as limited by your physician.

Magnesium
A 2017 study showed that magnesium supplements can help with depression. Magnesium is a known muscle relaxant, making it perfect for those who have BPD as well as those who experience migraines, anxiety, and depression. The treatment was suggested after a 2015 study showed that people with symptoms of BPD also had very low levels of magnesium in their system. You can also consume magnesium through natural sources such as leafy greens, dark chocolate, avocado, salmon, and Epsom salt baths.

Vitamin D
If you're not getting enough sunlight, then chances are that you have a Vitamin D deficiency – a condition which is also associated with mood and anxiety disorders. Supplementing with the vitamin can therefore help with the associated symptoms of these conditions. In fact, studies have shown that around 40% of people in the United States are vitamin D deficient.

Of course, it may be argued that correlation does not equal causation, especially when it comes to Vitamin D deficiency. The fact is that people diagnosed with mood disorders are less likely to go outdoors – which is why they get less sun. If you think you have a vitamin D deficiency, then you should bring this up with your doctor.

Vitamin D can also be consumed through certain food items like mushroom, cod liver oil, fortified milk, and wild-caught salmon.

Vitamin C
People with restlessness, anxiety, or suffering from nervous energy can also benefit from an added intake of vitamin C. Since these are known symptoms of BPD, patients can kick up their Vitamin C intake to around 500 mg per day. Studies show that this amount taken daily can reduce anxiety and blood pressure. Another study noted that Vitamin C can also help

manage symptoms of Type 2 Diabetes. Vitamin C can be taken in supplement form, but you can also consume it through citrus fruits, tomatoes, dark leafy greens, strawberries, and more.

Cacao or Chocolate
Cacao is the plant where chocolate comes from and according to studies – both have the capacity to improve cognitive function. A 2013 study showed that the chemical found in cocoa can help alleviate symptoms of depression and clinical anxiety. It can also improve memory problems and increase concentration. Dark chocolate is the best source of these flavonoids as opposed to milk and white chocolate which has a high sugar content. If you want, you can also add a few tablespoons of cacao powder to smoothies.

Of course, those are just some of the food items you'd want to include in your diet for a better coping mechanism when it comes to BPD. Note though that your doctor will also provide you with suggestions as to what could be included in your daily diet to help boost your mood. Certain medications may be given, and you'll also have dietary limitations depending on the medicine. For example, grapefruit is usually discouraged if you take medicine as it can render some medicines ineffective.

Herbs that May Help BPD
If you're bent on sticking to a natural route when treating BPD symptoms, you might want to consider herbs recognized for their wonderful healing properties. Note that the herbs mentioned here haven't been the subject of tests so while they're alleged to have BPD benefits, it's important to still consult your doctor about their use, especially when taken together with other medications.

Yerba Mate
Originating from Argentina, this herb is a noted as a natural anti-anxiety, anti-depressant, and mood stabilizer. It can also help with fatigue and promote a person's mental energy. Typically, the herb is taken as a tea and helps create a happy

mood for those who drink it. In its country of origin, Yerba Mate is given to children in order to help with temperament problems.

Kava Kava
A popular anti-anxiety herb that also helps with insomnia and fatigue, the Kava Kava can trigger a mellow feeling after being taken. If you're going to take this, make sure your doctor has approved your consumption, especially since Kava Kava may be a controlled substance in your country. In fact, some laws list Kava Kava as an herb that puts a person under the influence. Some studies also link the herb to liver damage, which is why it pays to be extra careful when using this natural medication.

Valerian
This herb was dubbed as Earth's Valium. It's been used to help with depression, insomnia, and anxiety. It can also be used to help with pain problems – making it perfect for those who have self-harming tendencies. It's a fairly powerful sedative, which is why it shouldn't be taken together with other sleeping medications. Due to its potency, the herb should only be taken at intervals and the dosage kept low. Reports note that Valerian can also trigger hallucinations so be careful when initially using it.

Have a Helping Pet
If you love animals, then you might find a pet useful to help with BPD problems. Animals have long been trained to provide emotional, mental, and even physical support to those who are having problems with day to day functions. Service dogs are quite popular, but pets that help with mental health aren't limited to dogs. There are cats, birds, goats, and so much more. According to studies, animals can have an inherent and acute ability to notice emotional turmoil even before the extreme symptoms occur. Furthermore, pets can have a very calming effect on one's emotions. In fact, studies show that the purring

of cats is set at a frequency that naturally causes a calming effect on individuals.

Specifically, people with Borderline Personality Disorder can enjoy a better quality of life with a pet that understands their needs. Of course, you'll have to wonder exactly how to get a pet who can understand and meet those needs.

Some BPD sufferers reveal that their pets seem to naturally fill the void or take on the role of support. However, what if you don't have a pet now and want to get one who can offer you the emotional help you need?

There are currently associations that provide emotional support dogs or cats.
The official name for these pets is Emotional Support Animals or ESAs. While it's not necessary to have your pet registered, there are some benefits to having a legitimate and recognized ESA.

Consult Your Therapist
Start by consulting your therapist about the possibility of getting an ESA. Generally, a DSM-recognized mental health problem is sufficient to justify having an ESA, but your therapist's input is still important to obtain the benefits associated with having an animal for mental health support. For example, landlords cannot refuse an ESA – as long as it is officially recognized as one. If you adopt a dog without - even if the pooch helps you emotionally – if there is no ESA Letter to back it up, you cannot benefit from several laws regarding ESA's.

ESA Letter
An ESA Letter is a document coming from your therapist which states the necessity of an ESA for your emotional and mental health. It must be written in their official letterhead, dated, and signed along with the license number, date, and place of issuance. This is because the letter is good for one year and

must be renewed annually to obtain the benefits associated with legitimation.

ESA Registration

Registering your ESA can be done through the system, but this isn't really necessary. In fact, Registration will not give you any benefits as opposed to an ESA Letter. This is because a registration can be obtained even without authorization from a mental health professional – which is why your landlord or air carrier will not accept these if you want to gain the advantages of the law. Instead, you will need to get the ESA Letter specifically.

Adopting an ESA

The question now is – how do you adopt an emotional support animal? The good news is that unlike service dogs, there's no need for the animal to go through specialized training. Emotional Support Animals only need to be able to give you *emotional support*, which means that there has to be a connection between the two of you so that you feel comforted whenever the animal is close to you.

When adopting or obtaining an ESA therefore, you can go to your local dog shelter and find an animal that makes you feel better about yourself. An improved sense of well-being and comfort is the key here – so you can choose any one you like as long as the emotional bond is strong.

It's perfectly possible to get a brand new puppy as your ESA, but adopting is by far the better option. This way, you aren't just getting an emotionally supportive friend but also giving a loving pet a brand new home.

While no special training is required for an animal to qualify as an ESA, it is important to give the animal basic training. This is done to make sure that the animal behaves while out in public such as cafes, malls, shops, and the like. A well-behaved ESA is appreciated and actually helps the ESA Community as a whole because it gives the animals a good reputation. You don't want to be the ESA owner with a misbehaving pet that makes it hard for everyone else who has an ESA.

Service Dog and ESA: What's the Difference?
Aside from the fact that ESA's don't need specialized training, there are quite a few distinctions between service dogs and ESAs. To start with, ESA's can be any animal – whether a cat, a reptile, a goat, or even a fox. You have more options with an ESA – but there are limitations. Your local laws will provide a list of acceptable breeds or animal types that can register as ESAs. For example, birds may be allowed but reptiles may not. Service Dogs however are limited to dogs, but further regulations may add a limitation as to breed.

Another distinction is with the service they provide. Technically, a Service Dog is characterized as one when it performs a function or task that its owner is incapable of doing. Hence, a Service Dog can help with the groceries, push the button to cross the road, seek help during an emergency, and others. Their functions include tasks beyond soothing their owner.

Benefits with a Legitimate ESA
If you obtain a legitimate ESA, then you will come under the protection of the Fair Housing Act and the Air Carrier Access Act. Note though that these laws apply only within the United States, so make sure to check how ESAs are handled in your country if you reside outside of the USA. State laws also come into play as there may be varying rules and regulations as to how an ESA should be obtained, handled, and registered. Airlines also have different rules as to how you can take a flight with an ESA.

Have a Premade Plan
The National Institute for Health and Care Excellence (NICE) recommends that every BPD patient have a Crisis Plan. This

essentially means creating a First Aid Kit for BPD so that you know what or where to go in the event of an episode. For example, you can keep a drawer in your room full of all the things that make you feel good. This way, all you have to do during an episode is go straight to the drawer and pull out whatever item you feel would best help you through the episode.

Since BPD episodes aren't always limited to your home, it makes sense to have mental health first aid kit in your office and in your bag – thereby making sure you've got something ready at any time.

Do Not Isolate Yourself
Do not isolate yourself from the people who can be a source of strength and morale. While you may feel depression and anxiety, the fact is that isolating yourself can only make these feelings worse. Instead, keep a good hold on your lifeline through friends and relatives. Knowing that there are people you can turn to in times of need can go a long way in helping keep the symptoms at bay.

An Orderly and Stable Environment
Studies show that a clean and orderly environment can help individuals suffering from mental health conditions. A cluttered home can lead to a cluttered mind in the sense that you have to worry about so many things, or have a scattered list of priorities. Therefore, keeping your home orderly and clean can go a long way in self-treatment. Having a routine, a to-do-list, a set of rules, specific spaces for specific things, and even being able to divide big tasks into smaller tasks, can make it easier for your mind and emotions to wrap themselves around certain events. The occurrence of the unexpected can be a huge trigger – which is why by allowing for reasonable amounts of control and order in your life, you can avoid the occurrence of these triggers.

Chapter 9: Self Help Strategies During an Episode

Part of therapy is to teach patients how to help themselves in the midst of an attack. Imagine this – you're in class and your professor is in the middle of a lecture. Suddenly, you receive a text message from your significant other, telling you that she'll be late coming home tonight. For a person with BPD, this could easily trigger your fear of being abandoned. Anxiety sets in, your heart starts to pump really fast, and you can feel an attack coming on – what do you do?

Since it's unlikely that you'll have your therapist with you at that time, you now become responsible for your actions. What do you do next?

One of the primary goals of a therapist is to teach you how to handle yourself during these instances. Therapy usually creates step by step habits that will help you to respond to these episodes appropriately.

If you haven't met with a therapist yet however, or even if you already have – the following steps should help you to self-manage a BPD episode:

Have a Safety Plan
Your therapist should be able to help you formulate a Safety Plan. This is basically a series of steps that you can do whenever you feel as though you're close to having an episode. As you read a little further, you'll find some suggestions as to what can be included in your safety plan. In many cases however, it's best to have input from your therapist. This way, you should be able to discuss the pros and cons of different strategies, as well as formulate a system that's specifically targeted towards your unique situation. Since BPD can come with many complications, a Safety Plan that's built just for you can go a long way in stopping episodes or diverting episodes even before they occur.

Auditory and Visual Grounding Exercises

This is a type of grounding exercise that BPD sufferers can do during an episode. Grounding exercises in general are those activities that help with panic, anxiety, impulsiveness, flashbacks, and disassociation, as soon as they happen.

Grounding exercises work by allowing a patient to focus all of their attention on the *present*. For example, during a disassociation episode, you might have this out-of-body experience – as if you are watching yourself do things that are completely out of your control. Grounding exercises essentially help put you back in control by stopping the out-of-body experience and allowing you to get back in touch with what is happening in the moment. The beauty of grounding exercises is that they can be done even when in public.

As the name implies, auditory and visual grounding means making good use of your ears and eyes to ground you back to reality. To do this, you first take a deep breath and start paying very close attention to the things you see and hear around you. Even the most mundane and specific things should be taken into consideration. For example, in the above example, if you start to experience disassociation in class, then you can start visual grounding by doing the following:

- Take a deep breath and look at your professor

- Take note of what he's wearing. Is it a shirt? A suit? Long sleeves or short sleeves?

- What color is his shirt? Can you see his pants? What color are they? What about his shoes?

With auditory grounding, you listen instead of watch. For example:

- Your professor is writing on the board. Can you hear every stroke of the pen as it glides on the board?

- Can you hear the whispers of your classmates trying to talk to each other?

- Can you hear someone chewing gum or possibly tapping their foot?

- What about the sound of someone taking notes on their laptop?

- What about outside sounds – the breeze or the sound of passing vehicles?

The beauty of this technique is that it can be done anywhere and at any time. It's also possible to create the grounding visual and auditory sources yourself. For example, you can do any of the following to help you reconnect with the present:

- Sing or hum your favorite song

- Recite your favorite poem in your head

- Call someone. This is incredibly helpful – especially if you have a support group that is always ready to handle the call.

- Whisper a mantra you've chosen beforehand such as "I am calm."

- Play a calming sound through your phone.

- Watch any show that makes you feel good.

- Look around the room and identify objects that start with the letter A, then letter B, and then C, and so on.

- Play with a favorite game on your phone.

Upon doing any of the auditory or visual grounding exercise, you will start to feel as though you're going back to your body. You might become aware of your heart pumping really fast at first, or the rise and fall of your chest with each breath. As the disassociation stops, you'll find yourself relaxing and overcoming the episode.

Tactile Grounding Exercises
Next up we have Tactile Grounding exercises which basically refers to the sense of touch. It helps to have a familiar item constantly on hand that you can hold onto in order to help ground yourself. Following are some of the most common Tactile Grounding exercises:

- Grab an ice cube from the freezer and hold it in your hand while it melts. Your hand will start to become uncomfortable and then painful due to the cold. Once the pain becomes overwhelming, you let go of the ice.

- Take a cold shower and let the water run on your skin. You can also do the opposite by running a hot shower or a bubble bath.

- Take your favorite lotion and start rubbing it on your skin. Relish the feeling of the smoothness as you rub it in.

- Mist your face with water.

- You can also keep a rubber band wrapped around your wrist and snap it whenever you're feeling anxious or angry. The slight pain will help keep you grounded to the present.

- Put a piece of chocolate on your tongue and just allow it to melt. Enjoy the delicious taste of the chocolate as it envelops your senses.

- Keep a pebble or a small ball in your pocket that you can handle and play with when you're feeling stressed. It can be anything from a beaded bracelet to a unique coin, depending on your personal preferences.

- Stretch your hands as high as you can and feel the stretch of your muscles.

- Grounding techniques can also be based on smell. You can carry a bottle of perfume with you at all times and take a whiff of it when you're feeling stressed. Oils like peppermint and lemon can have a calming effect.

The great thing about grounding exercises is that you can be as creative as you want. All grounding exercises have one thing in common – they compel you to focus on ONE specific thing. Hence, any activity or mental process can be a grounding exercise as long as you manage to keep your mind completely on it.

Practice Breathing Techniques
Breathing techniques vary and are open to changes, depending on the personal preferences of the person performing the technique. A good basic method is to simply take a deep breath while slowly counting to three. Now, hold that breath for three seconds before slowly releasing it over three slow seconds. Repeat the exercise, allowing your mind to go completely blank, and simply focus on the motion of your breath. Doing this whenever you feel like you're losing control of your emotions can help to put you back on track.

Meditation
Meditation is an excellent way to properly control your emotions whenever you feel as though you're about to have an episode. Practiced daily, it also helps to reduce the risk of experiencing an episode when you're in the middle of a stressful situation.

Practice, Practice, Practice
Whether you've decided to try grounding exercises, meditation, or breathing techniques – it's important to constantly practice the self-help strategy you want to use. The more often you make use of these techniques, the easier it becomes for you to channel your thoughts into a single idea or concept.

The beauty of many of the self-help techniques given here is that you can do them even *without* an episode occurring. There's no need to wait for a trigger. When you wake up in the morning, take a deep breath and focus your mind towards a specific thing – whether externally or internally. Your ability to "jump" into a focused state can be honed through practice so that when an actual episode comes along, it becomes easier to push through it.

Self-Help through Exercise
Exercise is often viewed as a cure-all treatment, with many doctors recommending it for practically any health problem. The question is – does it also help with mental health issues? As it turns out, it does. Exercise – the physical kind – can go a long way in helping restore balance to your mental health. As science explains, the act of exercising can release endorphins, which are the body's feel good hormones, but that's just a small part of the role a good exercise routine plays towards mental health.

Before we proceed however – what exactly do we mean by "exercise"? Exercise, as a way to alleviate the symptoms of BPD, does not have to be a full-blown workout in the gym or a one-hour run in the park. It's enough that there's sufficient physical activity to justify a little sweating and a little pull on the muscles. Hence, even cleaning and gardening can easily count as exercises within the meaning of this book. In fact, according to the Anxiety and Depression Association of America, aerobic exercises for as little as 5 minutes in a day can help alleviate anxiety.

The problem is this – BPD symptoms on their own, are enough to discourage individuals from starting an exercise regimen.

Depression, a low self-image, and pessimism are some of the hallmarks of BPD – which means that people diagnosed with the condition can be hard to convince to start working out – but that doesn't mean it can't be done.

Later on in this book, we'll look closer into how exercises can help people with BPD, focusing specifically on the kind of exercises that patients will find most helpful.

Keep Emergency Numbers on Hand
While you try to avoid them, there will be days when you'll feel at your worst – to the point where you might even feel suicidal. If you find yourself in this situation – call someone immediately. Your support group composed of friends and family members is your first choice, followed by your therapist. In some instances however, you may find emergency help services to be the best option. In the United States, the standard number for help is 9-1-1, but that's not the same in other countries. This being a case, make a point of knowing the emergency numbers in your area. If your city or country has a hotline for suicide watch, then it's also a good idea to have this on speed dial.

Finding an Outlet
It also helps to find an outlet for your intense emotions. This is a self-help technique that is best done when you reach the Second Stage of an episode – specifically, when you're at the climax of an episode. As mentioned, that is the part where you experience all the intense emotions like anger, frustration, depression, anxiety, and others.

Now, chances are you're having a hard time controlling your actions as a result of those emotions. You might find yourself suddenly angry and start shouting at your significant other. Perhaps you're depressed and drink a whole bottle of tequila.

When you hit the climax stage where you are compelled to act based on your emotions, the best way to handle the situation is by having a pre-planned action to do. You want to find a positive or at least, a non-harmful outlet for that negative emotion so that you don't lash out on a loved one – or yourself. With that being said, here are some outlets that you can use:

When You're Angry or Frustrated
- You can start ripping up a newspaper
- Keep a punching bag that you can hit when angry
- You can listen to loud music
- You can go for a run or hit the gym
- You can punch a pillow or just scream into it

When You're Anxious or Close to Panic
- Make yourself a hot drink and slowly relish the process of drinking it. Smell the coffee, shape the mug with your hands, and slowly sip. Studies show that warmth can have a very calming effect on individuals.
- Recite a favorite poem in your head
- Take a warm bath
- Jump up and down
- Start to clean and rearrange your space to help you gain some control over your surroundings

When you're Sad, Depressed, or Feeling Lonely
- Watch a favorite TV show or a horror movie
- Take your dog out for a walk
- Listen to a heart-rending song that you love
- Write a comforting letter addressed to yourself

When you're Spaced Out or Disassociated
- Chew some ginger or mild chili
- Clap your hands or slap your arm to get that stinging feeling
- Drink a glass of really cold water
- Snap a rubber band on your wrist

If You Want to Self-Harm
- Rub an ice cube over the part you want to hurt
- Draw something pretty on the part you want to hurt
- Take a cold bath
- Put some tape on the part you want to hurt and peel it off
- Use some kid's glue and put it all over the skin you want to hurt. Let it dry and slowly peel it off

As with grounding exercises, Outlet Exercises are versatile and are limited only by your imagination. That being the case, you are free to choose whatever outlet you want to use or whatever works for you.

Having Silent Signals
It helps to have a supportive friend who knows about your condition and can help you through the tougher times. Unfortunately, it can be tough for some people to realize when a BPD sufferer is struggling with an emotion or going through an episode. Make it easier for them by having silent signals or cues that make it possible for them to distinguish your mood. This way, they can take the appropriate actions necessary to help you through the episode. For example, if you're not feeling well – you can wear a particular bracelet or fidget with a particular item in your hand. This can silently communicate your struggle so that loved ones can offer some much-needed TLC, whether that means leaving you alone for the day, distracting you, or preparing you some hot tea.

Expressive Writing
Expressive writing is a form of therapy that can be done on the spot if you're experiencing an episode. It simply means focusing all your energy towards writing about whatever emotions you might be feeling in a given moment. Expressive writing allows for two situations: (1) it causes physical exhaustion and (2) it allows you to maintain a mental narrative of your feelings and emotions. The physical exhaustion means that you won't have to lash out at anyone. There's an outlet for your negative

emotions so there's no fear of causing problems with other people. By writing down your thoughts, it also forces you to think about what happened and whether your emotional outburst is logical or not. After the episode, your written words can help create a narrative of what happened and how you can avoid the same situation from happening again.

Learn More and Look Beyond BPD
Perhaps one of the toughest things about a BPD diagnosis is getting past the label. Most patients who have been diagnosed can't help but perform obsessive research about the condition to the point where their entire personality is tied to those 9 diagnostic signs of BPD. Remember that BPD does not define your whole personality. You are still *you* and BPD is just one side of you. Therefore, it makes sense to look beyond the illness and focus on becoming a person who has the potential to beat the condition and have control over their actions. Reading blogs about BPD, talking about personal experiences of people with BPD, and generally exposing yourself to the personal stories of people with the same condition will give you a better insight as to how you can live a happy and fulfilling life even with the diagnosis.

Of course, these are just some of the self-help techniques you can use for BPD episodes. Note that this isn't an exact science. What may work for you may not work for others and vice versa. Hence, it helps to constantly evaluate yourself, find out what techniques work, and what problems you've encountered when resorting to specific actions. Talking with your therapist about it will also go a long way in building a system that can help you with day to day problems.

Chapter 10: Exercises for BPD

As mentioned, exercise is one of the best ways to alleviate the symptoms of BPD. It's an excellent self-help method that promotes general health – not just mentally but also physically. In fact, studies show that exercising is a Keystone Habit. This means that by simply adding exercise to your daily habits – all your other daily activities can be positively affected. You become more creative, energetic, motivated, optimistic, and more productive. You also tend to eat less.

Here are some suggested exercises or workouts that can help as a lifestyle alternative treatment:

Yoga
Yoga is a perfect low-impact exercise that engages the mind as well as the body. There are many different types of Yoga disciplines today and your choice depends completely on your preferences. It has the additional benefit of promoting lower blood pressure, helps with breathing, and reduces occurrences of anxiety. It is so effective in helping with mental health that some therapy centers actually include Yoga as part of their treatment program for BPD, anxiety disorder, and depression.

Swimming
Swimming is perhaps one of the best low-impact exercises you can do – especially if you love the water. Swimming promotes endurance and flexibility while helping you build and tone your muscles.

Walking or Jogging
Walking and jogging are safe exercises that you can do anywhere and everywhere. Exercise has extremely great benefits as it targets the whole body, and is obviously cheaper than going to the gym. The added benefit of jogging is that it encourages you to go outdoors and enjoy the sun and the wind

as you walk through a jogging park or your neighborhood. Studies show that walking not only helps reduce blood pressure but also helps with anxiety symptoms.

The added beauty of walking or jogging as your chosen exercise is the fact that there are multiple applications that can help you measure your progress. There are tracking apps that measure how far you've walked or how many steps you've taken during the day. This adds a sense of accomplishment to your workout and makes it easier for you to set a goal for the day. Done right, walking or jogging is one of those activities that you can easily turn into a habit.

Cycling
Cycling is also a great way to reduce anxiety, maintain low blood pressure, and keep your mental health in check. This is really a matter of preference as some people may enjoy cycling better than walking or jogging. The beauty of cycling is that it doesn't leave much room for thinking. When cycling, you'll have to be constantly alert, your mind taking in all your surroundings so that you'll be prepared for any eventuality. It's much like driving in that you have to make quick decisions – forcing your mind to focus on the present instead of dwelling on negative feelings.

At the end of the day, any sort of exercise will help with BPD. Exercise in itself comes with many benefits – not just physically but also for your mental health. Participating in sports can also go a long way in boosting your mood and limiting the instances of BPD episodes.

Chapter 11: Meditation for BPD

Meditation is perhaps one of the most commonly recommended self-help treatments for BPD as well as many other mental health disorders. In fact, many therapists today incorporate meditation in their treatment plans. This just goes to show how effective this approach can be to overall health.

Studies on Meditation
Meditation has been consistently studied to find out how it affects the brain, particularly Mindfulness Meditation or MM. Here are some of the benefits associated with this practice:

- MM helps activate the PFC part of the brain, which incidentally, has been noted to be low-performing in those diagnosed with BPD.

- It's also important to note that MM is not a stand-alone approach to BPD. This means that while it forms part of therapies, studies show that meditation alone is not enough to curb the symptoms associated with BPD.

- Studies have also shown that MM can help change the unpleasant sensation of pain, and curb the emotional reactions associated with pain. For example, it can help manage fear and anger that results from experiencing pain. It can also change negative thoughts often triggered by pain.

- It has also been noted that MM can help lower the production of cortisol which is a known stress hormone. It has long been established that stress can lower the effectiveness of the immune system, as well as trigger the release of inflammation-promoting chemicals. With MM however, individuals will have fewer episodes of anxiety and in connection with these, less instances of pain caused by inflammation.

- Meditation has also been shown to help with emotional health, specifically self-image. Individuals who practice meditation report having an improved self-image and enjoy a more positive view of their life. Two studies involving over 4,600 adults showed that there were decreased instances of depression after practicing mindfulness meditation in their lives.

- Another adjunct benefit of MM is an increase in self-awareness. This might seem unnecessary in relation to BPD, but self-awareness can actually help when it comes to approaching triggers and developing grounding exercises. Your heightened senses allow you to correctly identify triggers and therefore, effectively create a system that can help you to stop or avoid them entirely. Self-awareness also makes it possible for you to properly communicate with the people around you. This makes you more aware of what is happening in your relationships, how loved ones are reacting to your condition, and how you can best meet them halfway for a mutually satisfying relationship.

- Studies show that meditation can also help fight addictions. This can stem from the fact that meditation improves a person's willpower and therefore makes it easier for them to resist temptations. Note that one of the common problems associated with BPD is substance abuse. Hence, a developed willpower can give you the courage to say NO to certain temptations. One study conducted on recovering alcoholics showed that those who meditated had a better chance of controlling their cravings. In addition, they were better equipped to handle stress related to cravings.

Other known benefits of meditation include a decrease in blood pressure, better control over physical pain, the prevention of memory loss, and the lengthening of your attention span. There's also the fact that meditation is something you can do anywhere – without the need for specialized equipment. With that being the case, BPD patients have a much better chance of handling the symptoms of a personality disorder if they include meditation in their daily routine.

Major Styles of Meditation

There are two major styles of meditation. All other types of meditation essentially stem from these two styles. Your choice depends primarily on what meditation technique works best for you although later on in this book, we'll talk more about Mindfulness Meditation, which is the recommended meditation type for people with BPD.

Here are the two major styles:

Focused-Attention Meditation
This approach encourages the practitioner to concentrate all their attention towards a single thought, object, visualization, or sound. The goal is to overwhelm yourself with a single concern to the point where your mind is ignoring everything else. Your focus can be on anything – your own breathing, a calming sound, a vision, or a mantra – as long as you are able to completely focus on it so that all other distractions are eliminated.

Open-Monitoring Meditation
This method is rarely practiced but is just as effective. It encourages individuals to broaden their awareness by paying close attention to their environment, thoughts, and sense of self. Through this style, you become deeply acquainted with your feelings and impulses with the intention of better controlling them.

What Is Mindfulness Meditation?

Mindfulness Meditation (MM) is a technique that falls under the style of Focused Attention. The definition may vary from one person to the next, but the widely accepted concept is that it is a discipline that teaches a person how to stay in the moment. Say you're washing the dishes. While soaping up the dish, you can often find your mind wandering towards other things – like what other chores you're supposed to do after the dishes. Mentally, you're already planning what you're supposed to do next.

Mindfulness Meditation is all about stopping your mind from taking that exhausting leap forward. Instead, you practice living in the moment or being mindful of what you're doing at that very second. This may sound simple, but it's actually harder than it sounds. It takes years of practice to perfect the skill, but studies show that even small attempts can go a long way in helping individuals focus and benefit from the discipline.

How Mindfulness Meditation Connects With BPD

Mindfulness Meditation helps with BPD primarily because it encourages the creation of a skill that improves your ability to focus. We talked about self-help exercises in a previous Chapter, one of those being Grounding Exercises.

Have you tried Grounding Exercises yet? If you have, then chances are you had a hard time with them. You push your mind into noticing colors, textures, sounds, and smells – but the wayward part of your brain is pushing the "trigger" to the forefront. It's like having two different images in your mind fighting for the spotlight. In some cases, the trigger wins because you spend so much time struggling that it becomes too exhausting to fight it off.

Mindfulness Meditation is a discipline that makes it easier for you to *switch* your mind to focus. Practiced religiously, you'll have an easier time of getting your mind to concentrate on what you want it to focus on. The spotlight becomes easier to manage, so that controlling triggers is quicker and much more effective.

How to Do Mindfulness Meditation

So, we come to the million-dollar question – how exactly do you do Mindfulness Meditation? Techniques are flexible and give you the chance to experiment with different approaches, depending on your personal preferences. Simply put, you can find what works for you and stick to it – each time gaining the benefits associated with consistent meditation.

Basic Step by Step Guide for Mindfulness Meditation

- Step 1 – Find a good spot. It can be your living room, your own room, your backyard, or any quiet and comfortable room. It doesn't matter as long as you have peace, quiet, and comfort in that particular place. You can even go to the park for meditation – as long as you can confidently sit down and feel secure in your surroundings.

- Step 2 – Decide on how long you'll meditate for. The standard time is around 5-10 minutes, but it doesn't really matter. You will often start small and increase the length of time for meditation as you get more proficient at it. It is often said that the time spent meditating is a lot like sleeping. Your body naturally goes to sleep and naturally wakes up – leaving you feeling refreshed. Forcing yourself to "come out" of a meditative state will only cause disorientation.

- Step 3 – Find a comfortable position. Most meditation images show a person sitting lotus style. This is when the legs are tucked against each other with the hands lying relaxed on the thighs, or perhaps even stretched upwards on the sides. Maintaining this position isn't really necessary for meditation – but it is highly beneficial for beginners. The lotus position opens up the hips, straightens the spine, and allows for easy breathing. It's a posture that compels you to relax, thereby making it easier for the mind to focus on the meditation. In all honesty however, any comfortable position would do.

You can sit on the chair, lie on the bed, lounge on the sofa – as long as you feel comfortable. Make sure that you wear comfortable clothes as well.

- Step 4 – Close your eyes and pay attention to your breathing. Again, we're doing the most basic Mindfulness Meditation technique here which is why the focus is anchored to your breathing.

- Step 5 – Feel your breath. This is where things get tough and where most people have a hard time. The goal is to pay close attention to your breathing, taking into account all the bodily functions that go along with breathing. Take a deep breath and experience the movement of the air as it settles in your chest, with your body tilting upwards as you inhale. Your stomach grows taut and your upper back stretches a bit. Hold that breath for 5 seconds and then slowly exhale, feeling your body relax as the air moves up your chest and out of your mouth.

- Step 6 – Amplify the process. Some people have a hard time feeling the movement of their breath, so it helps to use some visualizations or a mantra along the way. For example, you can visualize a ball floating in front of you, just in front of your mouth. When you inhale, imagine the ball floating right up on your mouth and when you exhale, imagine it slowly descending to your belly or chest area. Stick to this image until the ball feels realistic in your mind. Holding on to the image can make it easier for you to concentrate. You can also choose to add a mantra to this. It doesn't have to be complicated. Just add a 1-2 count, 1 when you inhale and 2 when you exhale. Repeat.

- Step 7 – Realign if you find yourself getting distracted. Distraction is perfectly normal as you get used to the discipline. It takes monks years of practice to truly perfect a complete meditative state, so try not to be too hard on yourself. As mentioned, 5-10 minutes is the typical length of time, but you don't have to stick to this.

Instead, just allow your body to naturally move in and out of the meditative state. Promise yourself at least 5-minutes worth of trying each day, and practice will do the rest.

- Step 8 – Commit to it. Aim to perform meditation at least once a day. Pick a time that's most convenient for you. A lot of people choose to meditate early in the morning or before going to bed. Just 5 minutes of your time each day is inconsequential but will contribute so much towards your overall betterment. You can use a timer for 5 minutes if you're on a tight schedule.

Mindfulness Meditation Exercises

The Raisin Exercise
Perfect for beginners, the Raisin Exercise is aptly named. It involves providing participants with raisins, and then the facilitator asking them to pretend they've never seen raisins before. You now pay careful attention to the raisin, its shape, texture, and size, how it smells, how the skin responds to manipulation, how it looks, how it tastes, and how it feels in your mouth.

It's an exercise that forces an individual to look into the present, thereby avoiding rumination or thinking about negative thoughts that may cause a trigger. You'll note that this is a lot like the grounding exercises as previously mentioned in this book. Despite the name however, the Raisin Exercise is not limited to raisins. It can be done with any type of food or fruit, so feel free to utilize whatever product you want.

The Body Scan
The Body Scan is a technique that often comes with a guided meditation voice over. You can find this type of audio voiceover on YouTube, allowing you to choose from multiple uploads. As the name suggests, the Body Scan encourages you to mentally scan your body, one part at a time – as if you're going through a

really intense MRI with your mind acting as the machine. Here's how a typical Body Scan Meditation Exercise usually works:

- First, begin the Body Scan by finding a comfortable position. Most people opt to lie on their back, but you can also choose to sit lotus-style or on a chair. What's important is that you feel 100% comfortable.

- Second, close your eyes and start the meditation by paying particular attention to your breath. Awareness of breath is usually the first step in all meditation exercises whereupon you become aware of the movement of the air moving in and out of your body.

- Next, you'll be asked to pay particular attention to the tips of your left toes, and how the air feels against them.

- Guided meditation in a Body Scan slowly tells you to focus on different parts of the body. From your left toes, you'll be asked to pay attention to your left calve and thigh before transferring to the right part of your body.

- The guided meditation often ends with the focus on your neck and head. Before reaching this however, you'll be asked to focus on the pelvis, the hips, the abdomen, chest, arms, and fingers.

- The guided meditation will be helping you truly assess and become sensitive of those different parts of the body. There will be moments of complete silence as you enter a meditative state.

- Finally, the guided meditation audio shall slowly talk you out of this meditative state. This is perhaps the great thing about the audio as it slowly snaps you out of meditation after lulling you into it. This way, you'll be able to properly acclimatize yourself to a more conscious state instead of instantly waking up. Without a proper guide, you might feel lightheaded or dizzy after meditation.

Again, it's strongly encouraged that you use guided meditation audio clips to help with this. Fortunately, audio clips are freely available through YouTube. You can download them to your phone, put on some earphones, and practice on a daily basis. Guided Meditations are as short as 15 minutes.

Mindful Seeing
Mindful Seeing is exactly what the name implies. In typical mindfulness meditation, your eyes are closed with your other senses heightened to absorb information from the environment around you. With Mindful Seeing however, you pay closer attention to what you see instead of what you hear, feel, or smell.

Here's how it's done:
- Find a space where there's a view. The window is often your main point of focus as you look at the sights to be seen outdoors. Using a window is often the best because it creates a TV-like setup, allowing you to really absorb what's inside the screen instead of having a wide field that makes it difficult to keep track of all things at once.

- Start absorbing everything you see outside, taking note of colors, patterns, sizes, and shapes of things. Don't label them. Most people look outdoors and think "bird" or "tree" which doesn't engage a meditative state at all.

- You have to "see" without labeling. When we say you should notice the colors, that doesn't mean you should look at a tree and think "green". There's no need to do that. The goal is to "notice" without going too in depth about the details. This is a common mistake people make during meditation. They think that they have to "dive" into it but in truth, meditation is all about sinking.

- Notice the movement of the grass or the leaves, the ray of sunshine, the pace of people as they walk to and from the sidewalk. All the while, enjoy every breath you take – the expansion and contraction of your lungs as you settle into a relaxed mindset.

- Do not allow your mind to have a running narration. If you find your thoughts wandering or having commentary about past or present problems, it's important to stop yourself and realign your thoughts.

Mindful Listening

Mindful Listening is really a group activity, often done with the help of a facilitator and several people. If you take part in therapy situations, then Mindful Listening may be part of the treatment process. Here's how it works:

First, each participant is invited to think about something they're looking forward to. Sometimes, it could be something they are stressed about or keep worrying about.

Once you've thought about it, the next step is to talk about it in front of other participants. The stories will go one by one, allowing each individual to tell their story while the others listen.

During such time, participants are encouraged to pay careful attention to what they feel while talking and while listening to others talking. The goal is to experience thoughts, feelings, and sensations through each talk. You should allow your thoughts and emotions to become engaged and truly listen to what the others are saying.

Since this is a group activity, participants are often asked afterwards about the different realizations they experienced during the exercise. Common questions asked include, but are not limited to the following:

- How did you feel when speaking?

- How did you feel while listening?
- Did you become distracted? What was the distraction?
- What helped you get your mind back to the present?
- Did your mind judge while listening? How did judging make you feel in your body?
- Were there moments when you felt empathy? How did that feel in the body?
- What are you feeling right now?

The Self-Compassion Pause

This meditation technique is perfect for people who experience anger and hate towards themselves on a daily basis. BPD patients tend to do this during an episode or even afterwards. It is not surprising that some sufferers will hate themselves for having what they deem as a debilitating condition. The Self-Compassion meditation technique therefore helps teach you self-love and how to be more accepting of yourself as you struggle through this mental health disorder. It is usually a guided meditation technique involving a worksheet to help the practitioner take note of what is happening.

Here is how it is done:

- Start by recognizing your feelings and considering the thoughts and actions you have taken that led to this moment and these emotions. Ruminate over all the things you have done, the actions you regret, and the choices that you feel were made correctly.

- Next, place a hand over your heart – as if giving yourself a deep hug. Take a huge breath and maintain this physical connection with yourself.

- The next step is the most important: acknowledge the suffering. Most people handle pain by shutting it out and this is not the goal of Self-Compassion. Instead, the goal is to feel the emotion so that you can finally let it go afterwards. This is a lot like allowing yourself to cry so that after acknowledging and feeling the emotion, you can now move past it.

- Afterwards, you will need to practice self-love, compassion, and forgiveness. You can tell yourself: I love and accept myself just as I am. If you feel like you have made a mistake in the past, then forgive yourself for it.

Self-Inquiry Meditation
This method of meditation is done to help with self-enlightenment. It is usually a guided form of meditation, or one that comes with a worksheet, but you can do it yourself without any problems.

The exercise goes like this:

- Find a comfortable position for you. Take a deep breath and try to attain a calm state of mind.

- Clear your thoughts of any lingering problems. You want to get rid of the typical considerations or worries you have in your head.

- Focus your attention towards the feeling of being you. Who are you? How does it feel to be your own person? What are the things that make up your inner self? What are your motivations? What are the things that help you get up in the morning? What things do you truly want in your life?

- Be as honest as possible when giving yourself answers. Remember: you are the only one listening to yourself at this point and it would be a shame if you lied to yourself. Masking your true answers will make it harder for you to truly understand who you are as a person. You are probably asking: what does this have to do with BPD treatment? Meditation of self-inquiry can contribute largely to how you see yourself and therefore, how you treat yourself.

Five Senses Exercise
This method of meditation takes into consideration all five senses, as the name obviously suggests. It is a guide on how to practice mindfulness for beginners and may be used in any situation, making it perfect for people caught in the middle of a BPD episode.

Here is how the exercise is done:

- First, you notice five things you can see. Look around you and pick five different things that you normally do not pay attention to. For example, it could be a crack in the concrete, a bent branch, or a wilting flower.

- Second, notice four things that you can feel. It can be the texture of your pants, the smoothness of your chair, the softness of the cushion, or the breeze flowing through your hair.

- Third, notice three things that you can hear in the background. The birds chirping, or the sound of cars, or the sound of the air conditioner humming.

- Fourth, notice two things that you can smell. These are the smells you usually ignore or filter out. This can be tougher since studies show that if you get used to a particular smell, you tend to phase it out. Pay close attention. It can be the fresh scent of the air, the musky scent of summer, the salty wind from the sea, or just the smell of fresh flowers in the wind.

- Finally, notice one thing you can taste. It could be anything you can taste right now. Perhaps you are holding a drink, so take a sip out of that. Maybe you are chewing gum so relish that flavor in your mouth. You can also just pay attention to the taste you are feeling right now in your mouth.

Mindfulness-Based Eating Awareness (MB-EAT)
Developed by psychologist Jean Kristeller, this mindfulness technique is specially designed for those who suffer from an emotional eating disorder which is a common co-occurring condition with BPD. The whole point of the exercise is to make people more aware of their eating habits. People who have emotional eating disorders tend to eat without really registering how much they managed to consume.

The therapy itself is more extensive in that it also guides participants towards healthier eating options and discusses the many health risks associated with improper eating behavior.

Practicing mindfulness-based eating awareness involves being aware of what you eat, how you eat, and how you feel during and after eating. It combines the use of all senses.

For example, here is how it can be done:

- Start by contemplating how much food you actually need by slowly, carefully, and deliberately spooning portions onto your plate.

- Do not dive in directly on your food. Instead, use all your five senses to slowly savor the dishes. Look at your food first, perhaps moving it around with your fork in order to get a sense of its texture. Notice the shape and color of the food, the various textures of the serving, and the sheer size of it as it occupies the plate.

- Next, take a good whiff of the food. What does it smell like? What are the flavors you can identify through the mere smell of the food?

- Finally, take a taste of the food and identify the various flavors that burst in your mouth. Appreciate the chewing sound you make and the soft clink of the spoon and fork against the plate. Chew slowly and deliberately, allowing your tongue to fully appreciate the flavor.

- Swallow your food and feel how it moves from your mouth down your throat, before it finally settles in your stomach. Acknowledge the heavy feeling in your tummy as the food slowly disappears from your plate.

Mindfulness for Depression
People with BPD are more likely to suffer from depression, which is why it helps to practice meditation specifically to target episodes of depression. Performing this exercise can reduce instances of depression, as well as decrease the symptoms associated with the condition. Here is what you should know about practicing mindfulness for depression:

- This exercise is called *Sorting Boxes,* and it starts with focusing on your breathing first. There is no need to control or change the pattern of your breathing into an even cycle. You just need to focus on it by being aware of each inhale and exhale.

- Notice any thoughts, emotions, or sensations that flicker through your mind.

- Now, imagine that there are three boxes sitting in your mind. These boxes are named: thoughts, sensations, and emotions.

- As you start to become aware of the thoughts, emotions, and sensations you have, metaphorically place them inside the boxes. Identify what you feel or think, and slide them into the corresponding boxes.

This exercise works because you are essentially tidying up your mind by putting the different emotions and sensations into their respective boxes.

Mindfulness Techniques for Anger
Anger is a tough emotion to control and can be destructive if allowed free reign. There are several mindfulness techniques that can help discharge chronic anger in a healthy and non-destructive way. Here is the most popular technique of them all:

- Start by sitting down in a comfortable position, keeping your eyes closed and allowing your whole body to relax.

- Draw in a deep breath, taking careful notice of the place you are in. Since your eyes are closed at this time, take note of how your body is touching the floor or chair, how your spine feels in this position, and how your legs feel rested against the surface of the material.

- Slowly let your breath out, thinking back to the time when you last experienced anger. It should be a moment where you felt a spark of anger, but the anger was not properly vented out.

- Now, this is your time to experience that anger. Recall the reason for the anger and allow your body to truly experience the anger. Feel your hands clench, your throat tighten, and the pounding of your heart to speed up in a classic sign of anger. Only upon feeling these things can you allow these same sensations to pass.

- Now comes the most difficult step: you need to bring compassion to the anger. How do you do this? You start by accepting anger as a natural human emotion. It is not exclusive to you, and feeling anger does not make you a bad person but instead, it makes you perfectly normal.

- Say goodbye to your anger. It helps if you create a visual image representing your anger. It could be a red ball, a flaring flame of flowers, or any other picture you associate with anger. As you say goodbye to the anger, you allow the image to fade away, piece by piece until it goes away completely.

- Gradually bring your attention back to the present, focusing on the rise and fall of your chest as you take a breath. You may feel tired and this is completely normal. Take the few minutes to rest and recover from the process.

- Finally, reflect on the experience. Notice the sensations that occurred in your body before, during, and after the exercise. Did you feel better after letting go of the anger?

You can repeat this exercise as many times as you deem necessary, or until you get the hang of it. At first, the whole process can be quite difficult, especially if you are not used to basic meditation. Once you become used to the technique, you will find it easier to control and direct your anger properly.

Chapter 12: Borderline Personality Disorder at Work and School

People with BPD often struggle in all aspects of life including work, school, and their personal relationships. So far in this book, we have talked about how you, as a loved one, can help a person with BPD. However, what if you work with someone, employ someone, or are teaching someone diagnosed with BPD?

We will tackle this in a structured manner, taking into consideration all of the parties in play.

If You're an Employee with BPD
If you've been diagnosed with BPD or suspect that you have BPD, you are not compelled to inform your employers about the condition. Your decision will really depend on the level of comfort you have in your workspace. Do you trust the people in your workplace to provide the kind of help and support you need?

To reiterate, here are the different rights you have as a person with BPD:

- The right to have your privacy protected
- The right to treatment with dignity and respect
- The right to receive services appropriate for your age and culture
- The right to understand the different treatment options available to you
- The right to get care that doesn't discriminate because of age, race, or the type of illness

If You're the Employer to a Borderline Person

If you happen to employ someone or be the boss of a person with Borderline Personality Disorder, understand that it's perfectly reasonable for you to become frustrated with how things stand. People with BPD can be quite erratic in the workplace, but if you meet them halfway, then you should be able to get satisfactory job results while still meeting the person's emotional needs.

Here are some things to keep in mind:

Inquire as to the Possibility of Mental Health Problems
Often one of the biggest hurdles for someone with BPD is finding the courage to tell their employer that they have been diagnosed with the condition. There are typically two different situations that may come in to play: first, your employee is aware of the disorder and is reluctant to tell you, or second, they are unaware of a disorder but have shown behavior that indicates the disorder.

If it is the first one, employers should be able to create a sense of security for the person in order to encourage him into divulging the condition. It is only after it has been acknowledged that steps can be taken to treat it. Hence, employers are encouraged to support and assure their employees that help will be provided instead of termination.

If the situation you find yourself in is the second one, it makes sense to gently nudge your employee towards seeking a diagnosis. An assurance that the company will be able to help is important. Many employees deny or are reluctant to undergo diagnosis because they are afraid that they will lose their job over it.

Find Out the Law and Company Rules about BPD
While you might want to extend as much help as possible to your Borderline Personality employee, you'll be limited by the law imposed in your State, This may further be limited by the

by laws or regulations of the company you're working in. For this reason, it's a good idea to figure out exactly what these limitations are.

Set Boundaries
The line between personal and professional can become easily blurred if you have an employee with BPD. As mentioned, there are laws in place that prevent discrimination among those who have mental health conditions, but that doesn't mean that you are completely devoid of rights as an employer. When broaching the subject, make sure to set boundaries in the office. What are the acceptable activities within the office? Episodes in the office are obviously not ideal, but what options does the Borderline Personality person have should they feel themselves nearing an episode? These are situations that you can tackle with your employee to keep the working environment peaceful.

Change Large Jobs in to Smaller Tasks
Another good approach is to take big tasks and turn them into smaller ones. Divide the big tasks into small bite-size pieces that your employee can easily handle. A huge task can be quite overwhelming, not to mention it can discourage more than encourage. The beauty of dividing the large job into smaller ones is that you can also create a quick achievement system. Each small task accomplished fosters a feeling of positivity and achievement – which contributes greatly to a person's self-esteem. This technique isn't just effective for people with BPD – it can also help every single person in the team. Done properly, the approach could boost company morale as well as keep your people productive.

Develop Clear Work Procedures
Create work procedures that are clear, concise, and visible throughout the company. You want these procedures to be transparent so that when something is vague, employees can simply look at the procedure to know exactly what they are supposed to do. This removes doubt and anxiety on the part of

the employee with BPD, while at the same time reinforcing the values followed by the workforce. The important thing about this is to make sure that the procedures are followed by everyone, and all remains fair and is equitable. Keeping the transparency limits the likelihood of episodes, as well as reinforces the limitations set by a working environment.

Encourage Telecommuting
You can also set up a system that encourages telecommuting or that makes it possible for BPD patients to work from home. The added stress of being seen by their officemates can trigger an episode – thereby making it more difficult for BPD patients to adjust to their work setting.

Be Aware of Breaktime
Understand that people with BPD tend to feel a lot of pressure when they work – as if they're constantly on the verge of snapping. Now, this hardly fosters a great working environment – but that doesn't mean the company cannot meet the employees halfway. Sometimes, all it takes is being mindful of the law-given "breaktimes" for those who are working 8 hours a day, and making sure everyone gets adequate time away from their desks.

Encourage Attendance to Counseling
Give some leeway with respect to counseling and therapy appointments. At the very least, be flexible with how your employee schedules their vacation time or sick leave in order to guarantee that they can show up for therapy. While therapy is often scheduled on a weekend for those who are working, take into consideration the possibility that plans may change as time progresses. One thing you should do however is make sure that someone can cover if the BPD employee needs to take time off for counseling. If you're in a profession with shifting schedules, keep in mind the necessity to show up to counseling when creating a schedule.

Create a To-Do-List as a Guide
A pattern, or a to-do-list, should make it easier for BPD patients to perform their assigned tasks efficiently. A to-do-list prevents their emotions from becoming triggered as the list is concise, transparent, and predictable. They come in to work, knowing exactly what they're supposed to do and more importantly – how to prepare for that task. For example, BPD sufferers may appreciate being told of a meeting hours or even days in advance. This will give them a better chance of preparing – not just work-wise but also emotionally, especially if meetings tend to trigger stress. If you're going to use a to-do-list, you might also want to follow up on each item, perhaps putting a big check after each completed task in order to provide positive reinforcement.

Provide a Safe Enclosure or a Safe Space
Giving your BPD employee a safe space where they can regroup, and rethink can go a long way in keeping them productive in the workforce. It doesn't have to be a plushy space or a room that's created just for them. Instead, it can be a small cubicle or a spot that you've made available for them whenever they feel as though they're close to hitting their threshold. Now, this might seem totally unfair to your other employees, which is why some employers merely encourage the concept of a scheduled breaktime. This way, everyone can benefit from the perks while keeping your BPD employee happy with respect to their space and need for a quiet time.

Offer Sensitivity Training to Coworkers
It might seem like added work, but it's important to remember that those afflicted with BPD also form part of society. Coworkers may encounter other BPD personalities in their lives, and it helps to have a background on how to properly interact with BPD personalities. Sensitivity training can go a long way in ensuring that they can properly work with another person without hurting their feelings, causing undue stress, or triggering negative emotions. You can hire someone who specifically has experience with this to teach the class. Many

therapists also host seminars and run this type of training for companies.

Provide Routine Confidential Meetings for Feedback
While it might take up some of your time, it definitely helps to give routine feedback to help bolster morale within your employees diagnosed with BPD. A feedback system also helps them narrow down their goals, figure out any problems they may have, and allow them to correct these problems to foster future development. Confidential feedback meetings will give them a sense of direction as well as make it easier for them to meet the demands of their job. Perhaps the most important thing about this however is your ability to communicate as an employer. Learning how to properly relay criticisms is a skill that should be cultivated among the managerial staff.

If You're the Coworker of a Borderline Person
If you work with someone who has been diagnosed with BPD, there are two common reasons for how you became aware of this. First is if your coworker told you directly and second, if the office felt it safe to tell everyone upon the consent of the BPD person.

If you're a coworker of someone with BPD, there's not much you can do besides being there to listen and be understanding. If your office provides sensitivity training, then make sure to be present in order to fully understand how to act or properly deal with someone who has BPD – especially during an episode. While people with BPD are strongly encouraged towards self-policing, there are times when they might not be able to help themselves, or when they don't have proper control over their emotions.

Chapter 13: Helping a Loved One with BPD

If you're reading this book because you have a loved one suffering from BPD, then this Chapter is specifically written for you. Note though that you should also read the previous Chapters, specifically with regards to the definition, characteristics, and symptoms of a person with BPD. You should also have a fairly good idea of the internal conflict that occurs within people with BPD.

Now, if you're reading this, then chances are you: (1) know someone diagnosed with BPD or (2) suspect that someone close to you has BPD or some other form of mental health problem.

If you fall under classification number 2, then you should definitely encourage your loved one to see a mental health professional for a diagnosis. If they've already been diagnosed, then you'll have to be mindful of the diagnosis while interacting with them. Let's approach this per situation.

Signs Your Loved One Has BPD or Other Mental Health Issues
If you notice many or all of these things when interacting with a friend or loved one, then it's possible that they do have some mental health issues:

- You feel as though you have to tiptoe around them because they can easily become emotional. You watch every little thing you say or do because it can easily flare up into a big argument. You do this to the point where you aren't comfortable in truly expressing yourself and become anxious with every interaction.

- Your loved one either finds you really good or really bad with no in-between. For example, you're either "perfect"

- or "selfish". If you're not "the best" then you're completely "unfeeling and unreliable".

- You often feel like you can't win any type or form of argument with them. Anything you say or do will be twisted against you, and their expectations of you are constantly changing. This makes it very hard for you to keep up and give them what they want.

- You often feel as though everything is your fault. You are always blamed or criticized for the smallest things. On top of this is that you always feel as though you're the one who has to apologize. There's this feeling of being manipulated by their emotions, specifically the anger, sadness, depression, or other outrageous behavior. Sometimes, even their guilt can make you feel as though it's your fault that they feel guilty.

- Your loved one shifts from one mood to the next in rapid extremes. It seems as though these shifts are irrational or unreasonable and there is often no in-between.

Common "Fights" You May Have with a BPD Patient
One of the most common problems loved ones encounter are the fights. It's not surprising that loved ones will talk about how the fights can be exhausting as the episodes come in relentless waves. Accept right now that these will happen often, and they will require effort on your part to keep these fights rare in occurrence.

You'll find that in many cases, these fights are repetitive, or hit on the same problem over and over again. Here are the typical categories of fights you might encounter:

It's Your Fault Fight
The fight may stem out of something completely unknown or something incredibly small. In many cases, your BPD loved one may take affront over something you did – no matter how small it might be. In some cases, it can be as miniscule as staring off into the horizon or looking at books in a weird way. Your typical

response here would be to ask what's wrong or ask them what their problem is. Note that BPD's will rarely answer this – they know in themselves that the fight started due to some small reason. Chances are they'll sulk the day away – and you should let them. It's usually better to take a step back as BPD persons go through the tumult of emotions during an episode.

The Projection Fight
Projection basically means that people attribute bad feelings and behavior to other people when in truth, they're the ones who exhibit those bad feelings and behavior. The typical mantra is this: there's nothing wrong with me, there's something wrong with you.

A BPD person may choose to fling their own faults and insecurities towards you, as if you're the one who's actually feeling them instead of the other way around. This is actually a common defense mechanism, but people with BPD take it to extreme levels.

When you are being projected upon, the first thing you should do is recognize that projection is occurring. Shrug off the idea of negativity being your fault, and instead consider the likelihood that the things they project on you are the things they feel themselves. Only after realizing this can you properly decide what to do next.

Inconsistent Fights
Another common fight that can be incredibly confusing for the loved ones of BPD persons is the inconsistency of their reactions. It's a no-win situation because no matter what you do, you seem to end up in the wrong. For example, your wife might be angry that you failed to tell them you'd be working overtime. However, if you do inform them about your overtime, they might become angry because you're disturbing them during the day. BPDs can be consistently inconsistent and it can be tough to figure out what they're going to do next. Your best bet is to simply do what you deem to be the most logical or

proper thing. For example, you can still inform your wife of an upcoming overtime shift – but do it through an SMS message to make sure she isn't disturbed.

I Hate You – Don't Leave
You might also note how some BPD personalities can easily do a complete turnaround when it comes to relationships. You might have a huge fight one day, and the next day it's as if nothing happened. This can be a good thing or a bad thing, depending on how you see things. Most of the time however, it can be incredibly confusing as you never know where or how to properly approach the problem. This happens because people with BPD feel as if they're being engulfed when people get too close to them. The emotions become overwhelming – which is why they will blow hot and cold, and then back again in an effort to calm down the emotions.

Testing Fight
This is possibly one of the most frustrating fight types because again, there's no room for escape. It's tough to navigate because no matter what you do – you're in the wrong. During fights, a BPD person will often rationalize that they're just doing something to "test" how much a person loves them or likes them. Another manipulating sentence is "If you love me, you would do this." Now, you might feel like giving in, having this idea that once you "pass" the test, then the BPD person will stop. However, this is rarely the case. Instead, they will simply up the ante. For this reason, it's important to create boundaries as soon as possible and enforce them.

A Gentle Reminder
If you notice many or all of the situations above, then chances are that your loved one has BPD or some other form of mental health problem. If you have BPD, then please understand that the above-cited situations are things your loved-one has to deal with all the time. Hence, it's important for both sides to employ a give-take compromise in this relationship.

Since this Chapter is for those who want to learn how to work with a loved one with BPD, we'll talk about you. First things first – understand that mental health problems do not make a person "crazy" or "insane". A person diagnosed with BPD is still capable of making rational, logical, and reasonable decisions. That being said, let's proceed on to how YOU can have a fulfilling relationship with someone who has BPD, or other mental health problems, for that matter.

Take Care of Yourself First
The fact is that having someone in your life with BPD can be incredibly challenging, physically, emotionally, and psychologically. It is completely understandable if you feel as though you yourself are having a mental breakdown after being subjected to an emotional roller coaster day in and day out. You may find yourself going the extra mile every time, at the expense of your own wants and needs. This is a sure recipe for disaster as you will slowly grow resentful of how things stand. It's not uncommon for people dealing with BPD sufferers to develop their own problems such as depression, anxiety, burnout, and even physical health problems.

This being the case, feel free to sometimes to meet your own needs and attend to self-care. Meet with emotionally supportive friends, pamper yourself, and find a way to de-stress. You cannot always be on-call as this will only cause a burnout eventually. Have a life outside of the relationship – whether the person with BPD is a family member or a partner. It's not selfish to relax and have time for yourself. In fact, self-care is something you should do even if you're with someone not diagnosed with BPD.

Remember the 3 C's
Do not allow yourself to feel guilty or blame yourself for the behavior of a person with borderline personality disorder. There's a chance you will question your own actions and decisions, often telling yourself that "if" you just gave in, then this wouldn't have happened. Failure in treatment or any form

of relapse may not always be attributable to you, and you cannot hold yourself personally responsible for it.

This is why it's important to remember the 3 C's mantra. This is:

- I didn't cause it
- I can't cure it
- I can't control it

Always keep those three thoughts in your mind whenever you find yourself struggling with the guilt or the weight of responsibility. Note that there's also a negative flipside to this. If you constantly reiterate those thoughts, then you might come to a point where you stop caring about the BPD sufferer's struggles. This is a line of thought that you should be careful of because this can fester resentment over the person with BPD. Instead, you want to attain an open mindset towards a borderline person.

Join a Support Group
You can also try being part of a support group for people who have BPD diagnosed individuals in their lives. Believe it or not, there are groups specifically created to help individuals talk through the trials of having someone close to them diagnosed with BPD. A support group will put you in touch with others who are dealing with the same symptoms from a loved one and can therefore provide you some insights on how to properly handle different complications within the relationship. These support groups also show you that you're not alone in your problems and that there are ways to get around them if you are willing to power through the issues. At the very least, support groups can also help minimize the amount of stress you feel as you can find people who will willingly listen as you vent.

Accompany Them in Therapy
Of course, don't forget that you can also be officially part of the treatment process. You can volunteer to go with your borderline

person during therapy when it is appropriate to do so. This way, you can give your own input and perspective on things in the presence of a professional. Even as an observer, you'll gain valuable information as to the personal struggles of a borderline person. This should help you adjust your own perspective, thoughts, and actions in order to better accommodate them without sacrificing your own needs.

Learning How to Communicate

Communicating with someone who has BPD can be tough. It has been described as "aural dyslexia" by some professionals because the patient may hear the words but have a tough time with the context. There's a distortion in how borderline patients hear and express their messages, making miscommunication highly likely. This being the case, talking to a BPD person requires tact, an ability to properly convey your messages, and most importantly – a capacity to listen and understand.

Active Listening
Your ability to patiently and actively listen is perhaps the most important aspect of communicating with someone who has BPD. No interruptions must be made during this time, especially if the sufferer is ranting, raving, or in the midst of an extreme emotion. In instances when the person is trying to explain their thoughts and feelings to you, make sure to nod and show them that you are interested in what they're saying – and mean it. While you don't have to agree with everything they say, it does help to maintain silence and simply allow them to vent out their feelings. Note that interrupting at this point is almost never a good idea.

Know When to Talk
Conversing with a BPD sufferer should be properly timed. You need to be able to read the cues and find out when they're at their most receptive. While the fear of triggering an episode may always be there, the fact is that not allowing yourself to express your emotions can be a source of resentment in the

long term. Hence, try not to match them word for word when they're in the midst of an episode. If this happens, take it upon yourself to take a step back and to continue the conversation when both of you are in a calmer state of mind. Pursuing the conversation in the heat of the moment won't produce any positive results and will likely lead to a full-blown episode.

Offer a Distraction

Some Borderline patients are capable of creating a distraction or ending the trigger as soon as it appears. This usually takes years of practice and is not 100% foolproof. This is why it sometimes helps to have someone offer a distraction that allows them to ignore the trigger. If you've read most of the book, then you understand the main principle of creating a distraction. The idea is to stop them from dwelling on the negative by prompting them to focus on something else entirely. You may point out something fun, turn on their favorite music, put on their favorite show, make them a cup of tea, or just remind them to start their grounding exercises.

Focus on the Emotion

The tone of a person's voice as well as the expression on their face communicates so much more than the actual words they're saying. This is why when talking to someone with BPD, it's important to focus on the emotion and not the words themselves. You can do this by paying close attention to their tone, and their facial expressions. If you keep trying to reconcile the tone to the words being used, you're going to have a tough time understanding the message. Instead, focus on the emotions alone and act based on those factors.

Set Healthy Boundaries

An effective way of helping someone with BPD is to set boundaries or limits that can be followed by all parties concerned. Setting boundaries can make it easier for you and your loved one to meet halfway or come to an agreement about what is acceptable behavior. Persons with BPD can use these boundaries as an invisible line that will make it easier for them to navigate through work, school, and other day to day activities. In relationships, these boundaries can help add structure so that both parties can get what they want while still making concessions for each other.

Understand that setting healthy boundaries isn't just for the person with BPD – it's also for you. The only catch here is introducing the idea itself to the relationship, especially if this is the first time that you're broaching the subject. Before we tackle that however, here are some tips on how to set boundaries:

- Introduce the subject when both of you are calm.

- Offer reassurance even as you introduce the idea of setting boundaries. For example, you can say; *I love you, but I am having a tough time with your behavior. I need you to meet me halfway.*

- Setting boundaries should be viewed as a process. This means that while you may want to set multiple boundaries, it makes sense to introduce them one by one so as not to overwhelm someone with BPD.

- Never make threats or ultimatums – especially if you're not capable of actually carrying them out. BPD patients have the tendency to push through the barriers just to see whether you'd push through with your ultimatums. Remember that setting boundaries isn't just for them – it's for you as well. Hence, you shouldn't allow yourself to constantly adjust for their sake.

- Never allow yourself to become an enabler. Most people with BPD are protected from the consequences of their actions by their loved ones. Do not apologize on their behalf and instead encourage them to own up to their outbursts. This compels a person with BPD to become more mindful about their episodes and encourages them to practice exercises to help with episodes.

- Never tolerate abusive behavior. Remember that you can always walk away during an outburst and simply come back when things are calmer. Just because your loved one's actions are due to a mental health disorder doesn't mean the physical and mental toll is inconsequential. Self-care is important, otherwise you might find yourself resenting and giving up on the relationship.

Support the Treatment

As mentioned, joining a support group of people who are in the same situation as you can go a long way in helping you adjust to the situation. As an added way of showing support however, you can also become part of the treatment or at least encourage the treatment.

Some of the ways you can help support the treatment process include but are not limited to the following:

- Volunteer to accompany them to the therapist if it's possible.

- Listen intently to what the therapist has to say about the patient. A support group will give you a general idea on how to live with someone with BPD. However, the therapist can offer a more detailed strategic approach, depending on the actual situation of the patient.

- Volunteer to help with things for the days when they're scheduled to visit the therapist.

- Volunteer to be part of any treatment exercises that the therapist may require of the patient.

- Celebrate small victories. Acknowledge whenever your loved one has reached a milestone in their treatment plan.

Convincing a Loved One to Seek Help

People with mental health problems may not be so open to accepting the reality of having a personality disorder. This isn't really surprising considering how mental disorders have a stigma in today's society. It's good if someone you love has accepted and has taken the initiative to consult a mental health professional – but what if that isn't the case?

If you feel as though it is up to you to broach the subject of seeing a mental health professional, then you'll need to approach the topic cautiously. Many people with BPD may react negatively to the suggestion and even cut you out of their lives, making it harder for you to lend a helping hand.

Here are some tips for convincing a loved one to see a mental health professional for diagnosis and subsequent treatment:

- Start by telling them how you need to have an important discussion with them. Pick the time and place properly – ideally somewhere without any distractions or where the two of you can talk confidently and openly if need be.

- Approach with empathy. Start by telling them how much you love them and that you know the situation is tough on them. Explain that the conversation is fueled by the fact that you care about them and want them to have a more fulfilling life.

- Be careful with your word choices. Words like *crazy* or *abnormal* should never be uttered as they have a very negative connotation.

- Be prepared for a negative, anxious, or upset reaction. This is perfectly normal.

- Do not get defensive. Instead, focus on the emotion compelling you to start the conversation: *I'm doing this because I am concerned about you.*

- Ask them to give this to you as a gift. Say, you want them to seek initial help as a favor to you, just to lay your mind at rest. Getting them to agree to an initial check-up, no matter the motivation, is a success in itself. A diagnosis of BPD or any other mental health problem, should be sufficient to compel them towards seeking treatment for themselves.

- Help facilitate the process by recommending mental health professionals and even scheduling the time and day – but with their permission, of course. Do not make the decision for them or just "inform" them of the appointment you've already made. Instead, just tell them your opinion about particular physicians on the list and volunteer to come with them to the meeting.

- If possible, offer to pay for the appointment or even the therapy. Most mental health care professionals offer a free first-time meeting which should help ease the burden. The therapy itself however can be quite expensive so be prepared to work through this problem together. If you cannot offer to pay for the therapy, you might like to at least offer to share a fraction of the cost. You can also do some background research on their insurance coverage to find out whether the therapies are covered. The perceived cost of therapy is a typical excuse used for avoiding treatment – which is why you should have a ready answer so there's less room for them to decline.

Chapter 14: Borderline Personality Disorder FAQs

Is BPD a result of child abuse?

Childhood abuse is a risk factor – but it does not necessarily mean that all people diagnosed with BPD were abused as children. There's a likelihood that they went through other forms of trauma during their developmental years. According to studies however, there's a relationship between BPD and child abuse. Depending on which study you read, around 40 to 76 percent of people diagnosed with BPD report having experienced childhood sexual abuse, while 25 to 73 percent were physically abused. Emotional and physical neglect in children is also linked towards BPD development and in fact, may be a likely cause for the condition.

Can BPD be cured?
Realistically speaking, BPD is not curable, but merely treatable. Upon diagnosis, the main goal of therapists is not to cure the condition but rather, to control it so that the negative actuations, habits, or emotions of people with BPD are kept under control. This basically means that episodes do not occur or even if they do, the negative repercussions are kept to a minimum.

Should I tell my employer that I have BPD?
Legally, people diagnosed with BPD are not required to disclose information about their mental health conditions with their employers. You might think you need to tell them, but this doesn't have to be the case – especially if you are able to meet the demands of your job. Some countries have laws in place to help people with mental health problems – such as the Equality Act. Under this law, there's no compulsion to inform employers of a BPD diagnosis – except for in special instances. Some professions are specifically required to divulge this information, primarily because of the delicate nature of the job at hand.

It's important to note that while a BPD diagnosis is acknowledged and may afford sufferers some leeway in their work, employers must maintain a balance between maintaining respect and getting the job done. Hence, as previously discussed, individuals who are not performing their jobs properly cannot rely heavily on a BPD diagnosis in order to retain their positions.

Should I tell my teacher I have BPD?

Informing your teacher that you have been diagnosed with BPD is dependent entirely on you and whether you feel comfortable informing your teacher and your school about it. Parents of people with BPD should also consult their children before deciding to inform the school about the diagnosis. The choice depends entirely on whether you think the school is open minded enough to accept and accommodate someone with mental health problems. Some schools have excellent programs designed to help students with BPD while others don't have any. Depending on your level of comfort, you may choose not to divulge the information or at least, have it known to only a few people.

Should I tell my friend's employer/teacher that they have BPD?

Legally, you're not supposed to. People with mental health issues are protected by the law in that their privacy is assured. This means that BPD personalities have full control over whether their status should be divulged. Hence, if you have a loved one who has BPD and is struggling in school or work – you cannot solve the problem for them by informing their boss or teacher about their mental health condition. The only thing you can do is advise them to inform their teacher or boss if they feel comfortable doing so.

How do I tell my family I want to be tested for BPD?

If you're an adult capable of undergoing the diagnosis yourself, then telling your friends and family can be done later on after the diagnosis has been confirmed. If there are those you trust however, it's always possible to bring them with you to the therapist so that you'll have added emotional support during the tests. One thing you should keep in mind is that BPD is primarily a genetic issue. This means that if you are diagnosed with the condition, then there's a strong chance that someone else in the family has it. That being the case, honesty is the best way to go – especially if you are surrounded by strong and supportive people.

What are the laws relating to BPD?

The good news is that mental health problems are taken seriously nowadays with more and more of the population demanding representation in governments. This is why some territories like the United Kingdom have passed laws with respect to people who have BPD and other mental health conditions.

Obviously, laws may vary depending on the country in which you're located. In the United Kingdom, there's the Equality Act of 2010 which essentially prohibits the discrimination by employers against people diagnosed with mental health disabilities. Under this law, employers are mandated to make reasonable adjustments to better aid the sufferer in their work environment.

Note that this sounds great in theory but not in practice. Discrimination is often present and can be hard, expensive, and lengthy to prove. Employers naturally seek out employees who are physically and mentally healthy because this equates to productive and quality of work. This is why people with BPD should at the same time, do their best to overcome symptoms through proper treatment.

Following are the different laws in force in the United States. Different laws may exist in your country if you're located outside of the USA:

- Americans with Disabilities Act. This law protects those who have both physical and mental disabilities with respect to employment as well as associated services. It aims to prevent the discrimination of people with disabilities in different aspects of life such as work, public accommodations, commercial business, public transportation, and government services.

- Civil Rights of Institutionalized Persons Act. This is a law passed by the US Government which aims to hold government institutions responsible and accountable when it comes to the care of persons with disabilities. They monitor these facilities to make sure that the people relying on these services are well cared for and get the quality of care they deserve.

- Fair Housing Amendment Act. This law makes it illegal to discriminate against people on the basis of their disability. It states that landlords or those who rent out houses must make reasonable concessions to those who have disabilities.

- Individuals with Disabilities Education Act. This law is designed to help those who have a hard time in school due to their disabilities. The act aims to promote a situation where disabled children can get quality education through an accommodating public school system.

What are the groups or associations that can help me with my BPD?

The good news is that BPD is known well enough that there are numerous organizations dedicated towards its treatment and helping sufferers adjust to a life with BPD. Following are the organizations you can look up if you want to get in touch with like-minded individuals:

National Education Alliance for Borderline Personality Disorder
Abbreviated as NEA-BPD, their mission is to raise public awareness and provide educational information for BPD sufferers and their loved ones. They promote research towards BPD while at the same time conducting meet ups to help those who are affected by this medical condition.

National Alliance on Mental Illness
Founded as early as 1979, this particular association is the nation's largest group that speaks for those who are mentally handicapped. Their main mission is to help with the improvement of the life of those suffering from serious mental problems, including the families of those people.

Borderline Personality Disorder Demystified
This is an excellent website dedicated towards BPD sufferers, specifically. It provides exhaustive information about the condition as well as the various treatments you can use.

Behavioral Tech LLC
Founded by Dr. Marsha Lineham who has BPD herself, this association trains mental health providers in working with those diagnosed with BPD as well as other mental health problems. They cater primarily towards mental health professionals who want to learn new possible treatments and to apply them within a controlled and practiced setting.

National Institute of Mental Health
This is the primary Federal Agency concerned with the research of behavioral disorders. It actually forms part of the National Institutes of Health and takes part in strategic planning on

mental health problems, priority-setting for those affected, and conducting necessary research.

Borderline Personality Disorder Resource Center
Located at New York-Presbyterian Hospital, this center was specifically built for those who are affected by borderline personality disorder. It posts current information about BPD, sources of available treatment, and helps those diagnosed to learn more about the condition.

National Alliance for Research on Schizophrenia and Depression
This is an alliance that accepts donations towards discoveries of treatment for people suffering from mental health disorders. As the name suggests, it is not exclusive to BPD sufferers, but it is fairly inclusive in that it helps address multiple mental health problems and their associated conditions.

Can you have both BPD and narcissistic personality disorder?

Yes. As already mentioned, narcissistic personality disorder is a common co-occurring mental health condition with BPD. It is primarily seen in people who fall within the high functioning spectrum of BPD. Usually, persons who refuse treatment are the ones who have, or are at risk of having, NPD.

Can BPD get worse if left untreated?

A straight answer would be YES, Borderline Personality Disorder can get worse if left without treatment. BPD is a condition that is primarily manifested through a person's actions, temperament, and life choices. When left untreated, an individual with BPD can easily burn their bridges – destroying their relationships with friends, family, and coworkers. They may have a hard time at their jobs, suffer through financial problems, and essentially go through one crisis after another. Simply put, the common complications may become prevalent and so ingrained in a person's life that treatment will require a more targeted approach. This is why it's important to undergo treatment as soon as a diagnosis is made. This way, there are less chances for bad habits to form, making it easier for a BPD patient to develop good habits, and keep their symptoms under control.

Chapter 15: Can People with BPD Succeed in Life?

After reading all of this information, you're probably wondering – can I still succeed in life with BPD? The typical mindset is that people diagnosed with mental health disorders – like BPD – cannot succeed in life. While they can definitely function, this might not be enough for them to lead a normal lifestyle.

But this is wrong.

In this chapter, we've compiled a list of people who have been diagnosed with BPD but have still managed to rise above the condition and make a success of their lives.

Darrell Hammond
If you watch Saturday Night Live, then you've probably seen this guy. He was a mainstay during the years 1995 to 2009 and once held the record for the longest consecutive tenure on SNL. He has impersonated more than 100 people on the show, but is best known for impersonating Al Gore, Donald Trump, and Bill Clinton. In 2014, he became SNL's announcer where he also appeared, taking on some of his most famous impersonations. His diagnosis of BPD was revealed during a 2011 interview with CNN where Hammond revealed that he was abused as a child by his mother. His coping mechanism was cutting, leading to a point where he was hospitalized. Aside from BPD, he was also diagnosed with Bipolar and Schizophrenia. In the same interview, he reveals that he was medicated during his time on SNL, even cutting himself backstage and being brought to the psychiatric ward. Today however, Hammond is definitely viewed as one of the more successful comedians of his era.

Susanna Kaysen
Kaysen was diagnosed with Borderline Personality Disorder at McLean Hospital in the year 1967 where she stayed for 18 months. Her fame came from the successful reception of her

book 'Girl, Interrupted' which was turned into a movie starring Winona Ryder. Parts of the book were actually inspired by her time in the psychiatric ward.

Peter Michael Davidson

Davidson is an American actor and comedian appearing on Saturday Night Live as a regular cast member. He was diagnosed with Crohn's Disease in his teens and was abusing medical marijuana to relieve the pain. Davidson had a hard time in his personal life which he originally attributed to marijuana use, but he later found out that this was because of his borderline personality disorder.

Brandon Marshall

Marshall is an American football wide receiver originally drafted by the Denver Broncos. He also played for the Chicago Bears, the Miami Dolphins, the New York Giants, the New York Jets, and the Seattle Seahawks. It was in 2011 that he announced a diagnosis of Borderline Personality Disorder for which he is now undergoing treatment. He also became part of a campaign dubbed "Who Can Relate" together with the University of Michigan, targeted towards national mental health awareness.

William Woodard Self

Born in 1961, Self is an English author, political commentator, journalist, and a television personality. He authored a total of eleven novels, not to mention five non-fiction books. A successful author, his work has been translated to 22 different languages. He also contributes to several publications including The New York Times, the London Review of Books, Harpers, and the Guardian. He's also been known to contribute to BBC Radio 4.

Vincent Van Gogh
It's hard not to recognize Vincent Van Gogh and his popular painting – Starry Night. Although a diagnosis of BPD during his time wasn't conclusive, studies show that he exhibited many of the typical symptoms of the condition. His Starry Night might be the most popular work, but he actually created more than 2,000 art works and around 800 oil paintings – most of which were completed in the last 2 years of his life. It's interesting to note that during his lifetime, Van Gogh was *not* commercially successfully, with his work only attaining the recognition it deserved after his death at the age of 37 years old. He committed suicide after going through poverty and suffering from mental illness.

So, is it still possible for someone with BPD to become successful? Of course. You'll find that there are many people who have managed to overcome the trials and tribulations of BPD to become successful in their chosen field. With the exception of Van Gogh, all of the people listed here managed to achieve success through hard work. Remember: during Van Gogh's time, diagnosing and treating BPD was non-existent. You are lucky to be born at a time when Borderline Personality Disorder is recognized and addressed properly through the help of professionals.

Conclusion

Thanks again for taking the time to read this book on Borderline Personality Disorder!

You should now have a good understanding of BPD and be armed with the knowledge necessary to begin treating the condition.

If you enjoyed this book, please take the time to leave me a review on Amazon. I appreciate your honest feedback, and it really helps me to continue producing high quality books.

www.ingramcontent.com/pod-product-compliance
Lightning Source LLC
LaVergne TN
LVHW011726060526
838200LV00051B/3037